Circumcision and the Community

*Edited by Ahmad Zaghal
and Nishat Rahman*

Published in London, United Kingdom

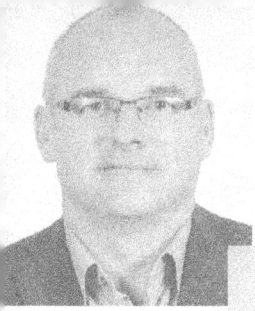
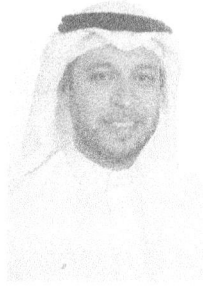
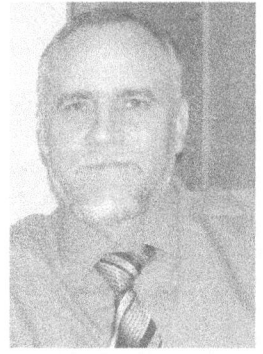
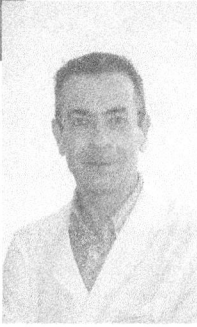
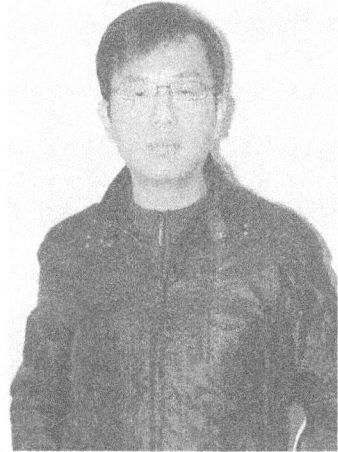
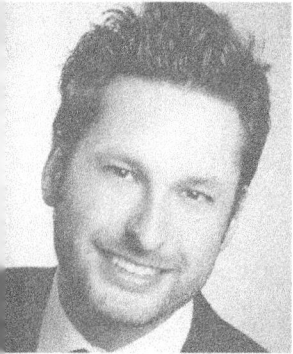
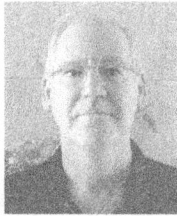

IntechOpen

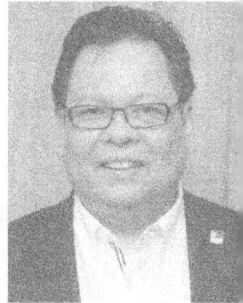
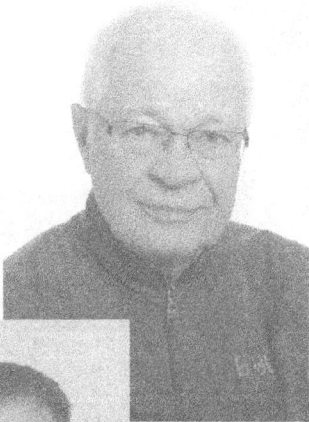
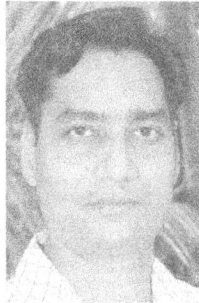
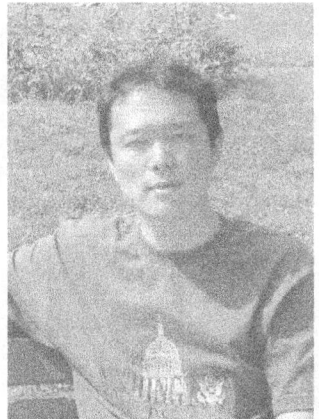
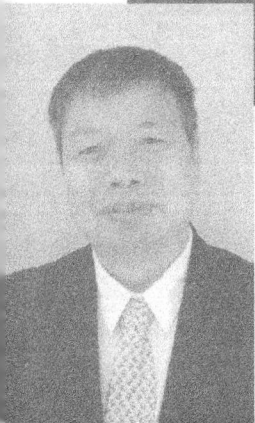
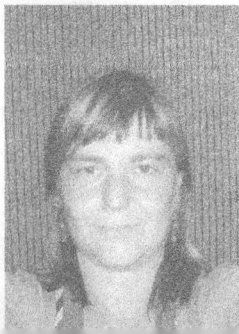

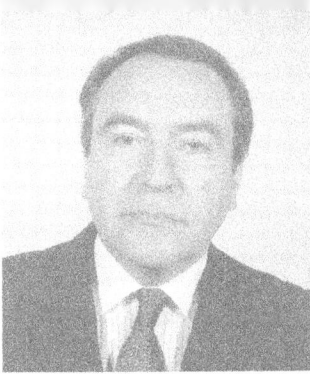

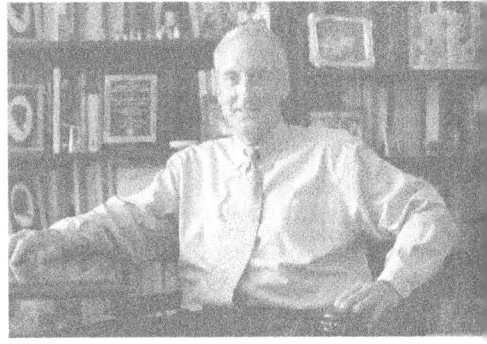

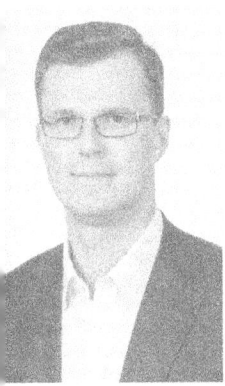

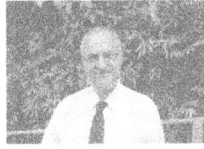

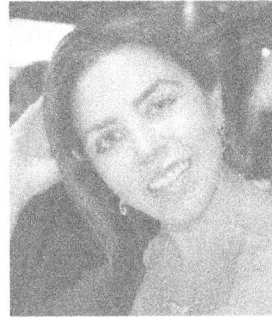

Supporting open minds since 2005

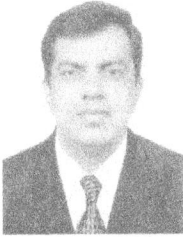

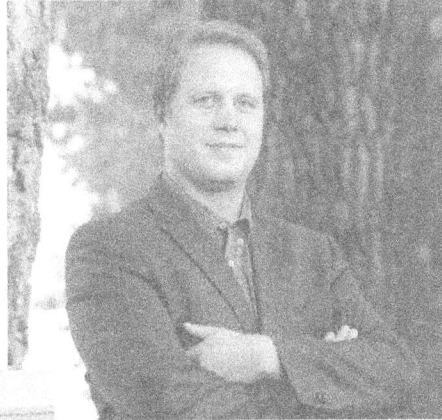

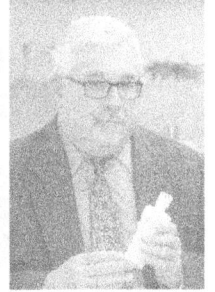

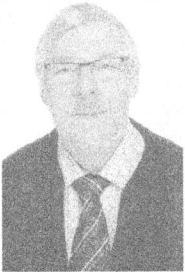

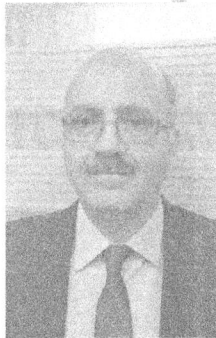

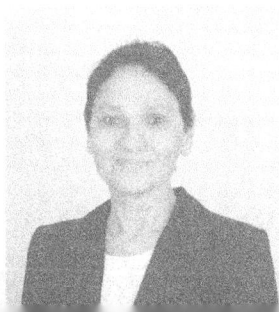

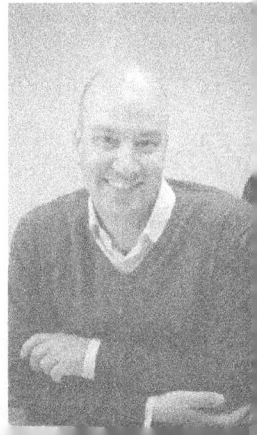

Circumcision and the Community
http://dx.doi.org/10.5772/intechopen.77815
Edited by Ahmad Zaghal and Nishat Rahman

Contributors
Lubna Samad, Shazia Moosa, Ozer Birge, Aliye Nigar Serin, Reem B Aldamanhori, Ruth Turnquist Mielke, Mpho Keetile

Notice
Statements and opinions expressed in the chapters are these of the individual contributors and not necessarily those of the editors or publisher. No responsibility is accepted for the accuracy of information contained in the published chapters. The publisher assumes no responsibility for any damage or injury to persons or property arising out of the use of any materials, instructions, methods or ideas contained in the book.

First published in London, United Kingdom, 2020 by IntechOpen
IntechOpen is the global imprint of INTECHOPEN LIMITED, registered in England and Wales, registration number: 11086078, 7th floor, 10 Lower Thames Street, London, EC3R 6AF, United Kingdom
Printed in Croatia

British Library Cataloguing-in-Publication Data
A catalogue record for this book is available from the British Library

Additional hard and PDF copies can be obtained from orders@intechopen.com

Circumcision and the Community
Edited by Ahmad Zaghal and Nishat Rahman
p. cm.
Print ISBN 978-1-83880-293-6
Online ISBN 978-1-83880-294-3
eBook (PDF) ISBN 978-1-78985-658-3

We are IntechOpen,
the world's leading publisher of
Open Access books
Built by scientists, for scientists

4,800+
Open access books available

122,000+
International authors and editors

135M+
Downloads

Our authors are among the

151
Countries delivered to

Top 1%
most cited scientists

12.2%
Contributors from top 500 universities

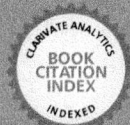

CLARIVATE ANALYTICS
BOOK
CITATION
INDEX
INDEXED

WEB OF SCIENCE™

Selection of our books indexed in the Book Citation Index
in Web of Science™ Core Collection (BKCI)

Interested in publishing with us?
Contact book.department@intechopen.com

Numbers displayed above are based on latest data collected.
For more information visit www.intechopen.com

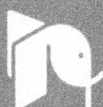

Meet the editors

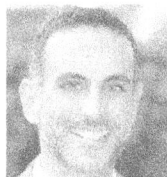

Dr Ahmad Zaghal is an assistant professor of clinical surgery and pediatric surgeon at the American University of Beirut Medical Center (AUBMC), Lebanon. After completing his training in general surgery at AUBMC, he completed a two-year fellowship in pediatric surgery at the University of Iowa Hospitals and Clinics, Iowa City, US; following which he completed another fellowship in pediatric surgery and urology at Chelsea and Westminster Hospital in London. Dr Zaghal is a fellow of the Higher Education Academy (May 2019), certified by the European Board of Pediatric Surgery (Oct 2017) and the Lebanese Board of General Surgery (Mar 2016). Dr Zaghal has published several articles in peer-reviewed journals, and authored several chapters on general and pediatric surgery.

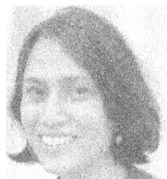

Consultant Paediatric Surgeon and Urologist Miss Nishat Rahman is a Consultant Paediatric Surgeon and Urologist at Chelsea and Westminster and Imperial College Hospitals in London. She studied medicine at King's College London and completed her specialist training in Paediatric Surgery in the London region having trained in Great Ormond Street, King's College, St. George's and Oxford John Radcliffe Hospital, qualifying as a Fellow of The Royal College of Surgeons of England in Paediatric Surgery in 2011. She gained further sub-specialisation by completing a Royal College of Surgeons Paediatric Urology Fellowship. During her training she was awarded a Research Fellowship from the Royal College of Surgeons studying bladder physiology. Nishat has extensive experience in paediatric urology and is amongst the few Paediatric Robotic surgeons in the UK.

Contents

Preface

The oldest documented evidence of prophylactic male circumcision comes from ancient Egypt more than 6000 years ago, as well as from other ethnic roots such as Sub-equatorial Africa where circumcision was performed on adolescent boys to celebrate their transition to adulthood. On the other hand, ancient Greeks considered circumcision an utter mutilation of God's perfect creation. The Judaism and Islamic faiths reinforced routine infant circumcision. Cultural circumcision found its way to North America in the late 1800s fueled by the fear of sexually transmitted diseases, cancer, and as a "cure" for masturbation.

The world remains divided between advocates and opponents of circumcision. Some have viciously fought against circumcision, whereas others pumped huge funds into programs to circumcise men in HIV endemic countries in an attempt to curb its transmission.

This book tackles non-medical male circumcision with emphasis on its relationship to communities and ethnicities from a public health viewpoint.

Ahmad Zaghal, MD, FEBPS, FHEA
American University of Beirut Medical Center,
Beirut, Lebanon

Nishat Rahman
Chelsea and Westminster Hospital,
United Kingdom

Section 1

Circumcision and the Community

Chapter 1

The Relationship between Female Circumcision and the Religion

Özer Birge and Aliye Nigar Serin

Abstract

Scholars of Arabic use the word "îzâr," which means defect, and the word "hafd," which means reducing and shrinking to express circumcision. Besides these, the words tahûr and tahâre are also used to express circumcision. European languages use the common expression female genital mutilation or circumcision to refer to circumcision. However, observations of some female mummies in Egypt and the description of circumcision on ancient Egyptian wall paintings supports the opinion that this tradition dates back very long and that it has continued for many years. The historian Herodotus states that circumcision was practiced by the Phoenicians, Hittites, and Ethiopians. Information obtained shows that circumcision is also practiced in the tropical regions of Africa, the Philippines, and by the tribes of the Upper Amazon and the women of the Australian Arunta tribe. The tradition of female circumcision that is originally a concept of the religions of African tribes has been associated with the religion Islam even though there is no reference to female circumcision at all in the Quran. Female circumcision is a violation of human rights. There is no legal explanation or excuse for persecuting women at young ages with various agendas like religion (!), customs and tradition or health in an area that affects their entire lives. This violation of women's rights can also be interpreted as a violation of children's rights.

Keywords: female circumcision, Africa, women's rights, religion, women's health

1. Introduction

Female circumcision or female genital mutilation has been defined by the world health organization as "all procedures that involve partial or complete removal of the external female genitalia, or other injury to the female genital organs for non-medical reasons" [1]. Although the procedure is called female circumcision in the countries that perform it, its negative physical and psychological effects have led to the use of the Latin term "mutylatio" that means to maim, to cut off (mutilation) in the medical literature [2, 3].

There is very little information about the origin of female circumcision. However, observations of some female mummies in Egypt and the description of circumcision on ancient Egyptian wall paintings supports the opinion that this tradition dates back very long and that it has continued for many years.

The historian Herodotus states that circumcision was practiced by the Phoenicians, Hittites, and Ethiopians.

In addition to this, information obtained has revealed that circumcision is also practiced in the tropical areas of Africa, the Philippines and by the tribes of the upper amazon and the women of the Arunta tribe in Australia [4]. The practice of circumcision is also called "tahara" in Arabic which means the procedure of cleaning. About the relationship between cleanliness and circumcision, the historian Herodotus asks, "where did the ancient Egyptians learn this, when the reproductive organs of all peoples on earth are remaining the same?". It has also been pointed out that cleanliness came before beauty for the ancient Egyptians [5].

The world health organization has classified circumcision into four different groups [2, 3, 6]:

Type I: partial or complete removal of the preputium and/or clitoris (Sunna).

Type 2: excision of the clitoris together with the partial or total excision of the labia minora (excision).

Type 3: cutting nearly all of the labia minora and majora together with the clitoris and preputium and sowing the edges of the open wound together leaving only a small orifice for urine and menstruation blood to pass (infibulation).

Type 4: is an unclassified group and comprises other mutilating practices (piercing, pricking, tattooing, scraping, cauterization).

Many applications have been carried out in unhygienic conditions without anesthesia and mixtures of plants, cow dung and butter have been used for wound healing [5]. Severe pain, bleeding, urinary retention, ulcers in genetical area, adjacent organ injury, sepsis and even death can be seen following procedures with scissors, part of glass, blade, bark, plant thorn performed by persons who do not medical professional training [7].

Infections, keloids, genital tract infections, sexual inherited diseases, especially genital herpes, increasing HIV infection risk, labor complications, sexual disorders and post-traumatic stress disorder can be listed among late period complications. Also, cases with Type 3 female genital mutilation are more risky since complaints such as requirement of deinfibulation, frequent recurrence, re-requirement of surgery, urinary retention, menstrual problems and painful sexual intercourse are frequently seen [8].

The symptoms of lower urinary system are frequently seen in females with Type 2 and 3 female genital mutilations [9]. Decreasing in urinary flow rate depending on infibulation causes urinary stasis and therefore causes repetitive urinary infections. Consequently, formation of urinary or vaginal stone can be seen [10]. In these cases, recommended treatment method is the deinfibulation. Urethral strictures or fistulas can be seen depending on urethral trauma during mutilation. In our case, urinary retention depending on adherences secondarily developed with mutilation was thought. It was observed that case urinated easily after deinfibulation operation. Cases with inability to have a sexual intercourse and therefore dyspareunia depending on improved vulvovaginal laceration and adherences in genital region after female genital mutilation performed in unhygienic conditions was reported [11]. It has been thought that genital mutilation applications increase infertility by causing sexual disorders (dyspareunia, apareunia) and genital infections. In case control study, it was stated that there was a relationship between primary infertility and female mutilation [12]. It was reported that psychological disorders such as secondary anxiety disorder and posttraumatic stress disorder against female genital mutilation could be seen [13].

Mutilation is still practiced in 30 countries in Africa, a few countries in the Arabian Peninsula, in some societies in southeastern Asia and secretly in ethnic groups that have migrated to Europe, America or Australia from these countries [2, 14]. Although the historical origin of this traditional practice is not entirely understood, there is evidence that it has existed since the ancient Egyptian civilization [15]. According to the reports of the World Health Organization, approximately 100–150 million women alive have been subjected to these practices, 6000 African girls between the ages 4 and 12 are subjected to these practices every day, and 2 million new procedures are performed annually worldwide [1, 14].

In earlier studies it has been identified that FGM is performed as part of the culture and tradition (like an initiation rite into womanhood) or religion, to make finding a spouse easier, or for reasons like chastity, genital hygiene, high morality or virginity [16]. It is known that circumcision is performed by Muslim, Christian, Jewish and also irreligious societies in Africa. In addition, no relationship was identified between religion and the prevalence of circumcision [17]. The prevalence of circumcision in Muslim countries Egypt, Sudan, Somalia and some middle-eastern countries has led to the emergence of an opinion that circumcision is a recommendation and a requirement of Islam. Sudan is an Islamic Republic that applies Islamic rules in social life and government procedures. Thus, religious rules and principles have an important role in the lives of the Sudanese people. The sayings and deeds of religious opinion leaders and imams hold a significant value in the eyes of the public.

The expression circumcision that is the subject of this study refers only to female circumcision. The tradition of female circumcision that is originally a concept of the religions of African tribes has been associated with the religion Islam even though there is no reference to female circumcision at all in the Quran. The differences between religious systems in countries that practice female circumcision show that circumcision exists as a cultural phenomenon in other non-Islamic cultures. In this respect, it is believed that the tradition of female circumcision in Islamic African countries originates from African tribes. The highest levels of the tradition of female circumcision practiced by some African Animist groups in the pre-Islamic era have been encountered in the Yoruba and Bakango tribes. In addition to this, it is known that it was practiced widely in the era of the Kingdom of Kush ruled by Black pharaohs in Nubia in Upper Egypt during the time of the 18th dynasty. While Islam was spreading among the Animist tribes of Africa, the tradition of female circumcision influenced some schools of Islam through mutual interactions. Leaders of African tribes that converted to Islam and wanted to continue the practices of female circumcision associated it with Islam. Consequently, a belief that this practice is a requirement of Islam emerged [18].

2. History and methods

The practice of female circumcision differs by country and can be performed at any time starting from babyhood until the ages of 13–14 [7, 8]. In half of the countries circumcision is performed in, it is done before the age of 5 by a woman called a "daya," usually without numbing the genital area and by using non-sterile tools like knives, razor blades, sharp pieces of glass or sharp edges of tin. Acacia thorns, bone nails, needles, strings made from animal hair or leather are used to close the wound, and then the girl's legs are tied together tightly from the knee to the hip in an upright position. The circumcised girl lies without moving for a few weeks and is helped to urinate and defecate where she lies. During the circumcision, apart from the daya, other women gathered around the girl hold the girls' arms and legs tightly, some press her shoulders down to prevent her from moving. To prevent the girl from swallowing or biting her tongue a cloth or stick is placed in her mouth, and the other women play the tambourine and sing songs loudly to mask the screaming [4, 9, 10].

According to the UNICEF report, around 125 million women have been circumcised to this day, and nearly 30 million girls are in danger of circumcision. Girls between the ages of 3 and 10 are subjected to this torture every year. Egypt (most prominently), Sudan, Ethiopia, Nigeria, Kenya, Indonesia, Malaysia, and Somali are among the countries where the tradition of female circumcision is practiced. It is rarer in Syria, Iraq and Iran and is also seen in Europe, Canada, America and Australia as a result of migration [9, 10, 12].

Our research revealed that female genital mutilation was used in past to treat some female disorders like hysteria, epilepsy, masturbation, lesbianism, sex addiction and mental disorders in the United States of America and west Europe [4, 13].

The social scientists studying this topic have separate views that support each other. Among these, there are opinions that female circumcision dates back to the Neolithic era, that the Egyptians used circumcision to prevent their relatives and slaves from getting pregnant and that it was also prevalent in the Arabian Peninsula before Islam [19].

Another aspect of the origin and spread of the tradition of female circumcision is the economic and geographic background. Harsh climate changes between Africa and the inner parts of Asia accelerated the replacement of the democratic and peaceful matriarchal society with a patriarchal society. As Nevâl es-Sa'dâvî has also stated, during the era of the pharaohs Egyptian women held important positions in the field of governing as well as religion. Research conducted supports the opinion that ancient pagan gods were also female. However, the period of goddesses dates further back than the origin of patriarchal societies and feudalism. Women in ancient agricultural societies succeeded to preserve their social and political positions. However, the advancements in agriculture and its evolution into a means of living led to the birth of private ownership. The rise of class discrimination and the developments disrupted the position of women and made them lose their prior prestige and reputation. They were pushed towards the lower levels in all of the hierarchic systems [20].

The works of Nevâl es-Sa'dâvî and Esma ed-Darîr on this subject have enabled access to first-hand reliable information and have facilitated raising awareness at a global level. Besides this, apprehension has increased with the development of feminist awareness and the international women's health movement [21].

If we examine the religious aspect of female circumcision here, we must say that it is not included in any of the heavenly religions. However, there is also mention of inauthentic hadith on the subject of female circumcision. In one of these fake hadiths, it is reported that the prophet Muhammad (pbuh) summoned a woman that circumcised girls in Mecca and said, "do not cut too deep that is better for the woman and more liked by her husband [22]. Besides this, according to a hadith narrated by Abu Hureyrah, the prophet (pbuh) said: The fitrah (human nature) is five things—circumcision, shaving the pubes, cutting the nails, plucking the armpit hairs, and trimming the mustache [23]." It is clearly stated that this expression does not concern female circumcision and that it was interpreted with bias. Those opposing the people that base this practice on religious requirements cite the Quran as a source for their opposing opinions. In this context they refer to the holy book that is the source of Islam and give examples from verses of the Quran (Surah [passage]:verse of the Quran; Furkan:2, Nur:115, Rum:30, Âli İmrân:6) [22].

One of the best arguments that female circumcision is prohibited in Islam is that the Quran and the sunnah (the verbally transmitted record of the teachings, deeds and sayings, silent permissions (or disapprovals) of the Islamic prophet Muhammad) of the prophet reject practices against human nature. In this context, female circumcision contradicts the systematic thought of the holy Quran [22].

The religious assessment should also include the fatwa (Islamic legislation) issued by renowned people and institutions of the Islamic community based on religious foundations that contradict these opinions. These are fatwa that state that female circumcision is legal in Islam and that its prohibition is unwarranted [23].

The continuation of the practice despite knowledge of its harms can be attributed to the culture and the associated emotional behaviors. When the condition is examined in Sudan, the country where female circumcision is most prevalent and where it is practiced in its most severe form, it will be seen that female circumcision is one of the most delicate subjects of that culture. In the Sudanese society where the pride of a family depends on virginity, being circumcised bears the characteristics of a cachet. In the Sudanese society, women must be virgins physically and symbolically, and this is possible with circumcision [19].

Although it is incorrect according to religious references, the opinion that women are a source of mischief and that they should be kept under control that is customary in Muslim societies plays an important role in the continuation of female circumcision in the countries it is practiced in. In a society where non-circumcised women are regarded as prostitutes, the highest authority in the family, the grandmothers continue this practice that is an indispensable aspect of their culture to them. Because it is a matter of honor and pride for the family they themselves deliver the girls to the dayas.

According to Nevâl es-Sa'dâvî, economic reasons play an important role in the origination and persistence of female circumcisions. The historical process shows that the oppression of women began with the evolution into a patriarchal society. The economic interests of society and the moral and religious values of the patriarchal system overlapped and gained support. Historical research shows that chastity belts, circumcision and other forms of violence were methods used to suppress female sexuality. It was aimed to restrain female sexuality and women were not allowed to experience sexuality unless it was for economic reasons. The daya and doctors that earn a living by performing these procedures must also be remembered among economic reasons. The fact that women in Sudan suffer this procedure multiple times due to reasons like marriage, birth, divorce, and re-marriage displays the economic dimensions concerning the practitioners of circumcision. It is known that daya are also required the wedding night [24].

The subject of circumcision is directly related to female sexuality. Together with the most delicate subjects of society, religion and policy, this relationship is more prominent in less developed countries. Girls that are circumcised are turned into targets vulnerable to physical and mental abuse without the capacity of thinking, understanding and judgment.

Cultural, social, psychological and economic conditions appear to be the major factors in persisting the practice of female circumcision. Esthetic concerns may also be added to these factors. It is also stated that the concepts of tradition and religion are also strong encouragers [25]. In addition to this opinion, many of the Muslims and academics in the west argue that circumcision is more related to culture than religion. Likewise, the authentic and apodictic references of Islam reject female circumcision. Accordingly, the philosophy of Islamic law (fiqh) only accepts circumcision of boys known by the name "hıtân." Unfortunately, it can be seen that the religion has been manipulated to express that female circumcision is a religious requirement in many countries in Africa [26].

Raising public awareness has a major importance in combating female circumcision. While the public is enlightened religiously and medically, the rights of women in this area must be protected legally through legal enforcement. The Egyptian Mufti Office has announced that they are against female circumcision and that this practice has no religious basis. Similarly, the Religious Affairs Administration of the Republic of Turkey also states that female circumcision is a procedure that the religion Islam prohibits. At this point, the explanations of Nevâl es-Sa'dâvî are important in the religious and medical aspects: Religion comprises the concept of health, love, justice, equality and honesty for all people, man or woman. Thus, a religion that desires to harm and sicken the bodies of girls and women is unthinkable. How could religion order to cut off an organ created by Allah? No organ or anything else is created by Allah randomly [22]. Islam does not allow human nature to be disrupted. On the other hand, male circumcision has been categorized as Sunnah and wajib (that which is proven on the basis of ambiguous evidence) on the basis of Islamic law and certain health benefits.

3. Conclusion

The importance of informing the public and education in ending the practice of female genital circumcision that has no religious basis and endangers the future of children and affects them is evident. Also, the society must acquire a high level of consciousness with the capacity to handle and resolve the problems of children to protect them instead of maiming them by circumcision. Families that want these harmful customs and traditions to come to an end want to enlighten the public and also demand laws and punishments that the whole society will be bound by.

Author details

Özer Birge[1*] and Aliye Nigar Serin[2]

1 Department of Gynaecology and Obstetrics, Akdeniz University Hospital, Antalya, Turkey

2 Department of Gynaecology and Obstetrics, Osmaniye State Hospital, Osmaniye, Turkey

*Address all correspondence to: ozbirge@gmail.com

IntechOpen

References

[1] Kiragu K, mutilation F g. A reproductive health concern. Population Reports. Series Journal. Oct 1995; (41 Suppl):1-4

[2] Black JA, Debelle GD. Female genital mutilation in Britain. British Medical Journal. 1995;**310**:1590-1592

[3] Female Genital Mutilation. ACOG Committee Opinion. Committee on international Affairs. No. 151. 1995. Available from: www.ncbi.nlm.nih.gov [Accessed: 3 May 2019]

[4] UNFPA is the United Nations Sexual and Reproductive Health Agency. 2013. Available from: www.unfpa.org/gender/ practices [Accessed: 2 May 2019]

[5] Cultural Survival Quarterly Magazine. 1985. Clitoridectomy and Infibulation. Available from: www. culturalsurvival.org [Accessed: 3 May 2019]

[6] Macready N. Female genital mutilation outlawed in United States. British Medical Journal. 1996;**313**(7065):1103

[7] Chelala C. A critical move against female genital mutilation. Populi. 1998;**25**(1):13-15

[8] Rushwan H. Female genital mutilation, working paper for UNFPA Technical Consultation on Female Genital Mutilation, Ouagadougou, Burkina Faso, 1996; and Toubia N, 1993, op. cit. (see reference 4)

[9] Extract of sample "Female Genital Multilation" WHO. 2012. Available from: https://studentshare.org/ sociology/1457960-female-genital-multilation [Accessed: 2 May 2019]

[10] UNICEF. Innocenti Research Centre. The General Measures of the Convention on the Rights of the Child: The Process in Europe and Central Asia; 2006;50. ISBN-10: 88-89129-42-5

[11] UNFPA. 2013. Available from: www. unfpa.org/gender/practices [Accessed: 2 May 2019]

[12] UNICEF. Female Genital Mutilation/Cutting: A Statistical Overview and Exploration of the Dynamics of Change. July 2013;184. ISBN: 978-92-806-4703-7

[13] Rodríguez SB. Female Circumcision and Clitoridectomy in the United States: A History of a Medical Treatment. 2014. University of Rochester Press. Available from: www.academia.edu [Accessed: 5 May 2019]

[14] World Health Organization. Division of Family Health. Female Genital Mutilation: Report of a WHO Technical Working Group, Geneva, 17-19 July 1995. 1996. Available from: www.who.int/iris/handle/10665/63602 [Accessed: 3 May 2019]

[15] Knight M. Curing or ritual mutilation? Some remarks on the practice of female and male circumcision in Graeco-Roman Egypt. ISIS. 2001;**92**(2):317-338

[16] Nour NM. Female genital cutting: A persisting practice. Reviews in Obstetrics and Gynecology. 2008;**1**(3):135-139

[17] Obermeyer CM. Female genital surgeries: The known, the unknown, and the unknowable. Medical Anthropology Quarterly. 1999;**13**(1):79-106

[18] İlkkaracan P. Women and Sexuality in Muslim Societies (Translator Ebru Salman). İstanbul: İletişim; 2006

[19] Hayes RO. Female genital mutilation, fertility control, women's

roles, and the patrilineage in modern
Sudan: A functional analysis. American
Ethnologist. 1975;**4**(2):617-633

[20] Es-Saʿdâvî N. The Hidden Face of
Eve (Translated by Sibel Özbudun).
İstanbul: Anahtar Kitaplar; 1991

[21] Gordon D. Female circumcision
and genital operations in Egypt and
the Sudan: A dilemma for medical
anthropology. Medical Antropology
Quarterly, New Series. 1991;**1**(5):3-14

[22] Sâmi ʿAvd ez-Zîyb ebu es-Sêhiliyye.
Hitên ez-Zekûr veʾl-inâs ʿındeʾl-yehûd
veʾlmesîhiyyîn veʾl-muslimîn el-cedel
ed-dînî veʾt-tıbbî veʾl-ictimâʿî veʾl-
kânûnî. 2012. Available from: http://
www.sami-aldeeb.com/sections/
view.php?id=18&action=publicatio
nsm21.01.2014

[23] Muhammed Ali S-BH. Hitên el-înâs
eş-şerʿî. 4th ed. el-Hartûm: matbaʿat
es-Sidêd; 2009

[24] Saadawi NEl. A creative and
dissident life. Infed. 2000. Available
from: http://africawrites.org/blog/
the-politics-of-health [Accessed: 3 May
2019]

[25] Essak B, Sailo E, İllahe K. Teşvîh
el-ağdâʿ et-tenâsuliyye liʾl-inâs. (FGM).
Helsinki, Tyylipaino: Africarewo ry
(African Care Women); 2011

[26] Von der Osten-Sacken T, Uwer T. Is
female genital mutilation an Islamic
problem? Middle East Quarterly.
Winter. 2007:29-36. Available from:
http://www.meforum.org/1629/
is-female-genitalmutilation-an-islamic-
problem [Accessed: 22 January 2014]

Chapter 2

Scaling Safe Circumcisions in Communities

Shazia Moosa and Lubna Samad

Abstract

Male circumcision (MC), although a common and simple procedure, is not available to a majority of the population as a safe, sterile intervention. The convincing evidence of the protective role of circumcision towards the spread of STDs (particularly HIV) led to the establishment of voluntary, adult male circumcision programmes in high-HIV-burden countries. In low- and middle-income Muslim countries, where the need for circumcision is high, there is an evident gap in access to, and delivery of, this procedure. Large-scale programmes aimed at circumcising male babies in settings where circumcision is a religious requirement, as opposed to a medical indication, have not been established. This chapter would draw upon current guidelines and literature, review existing programmes that have attempted to establish community-based safe circumcision initiatives and discuss strategies for sustainable scale-up to meet this huge public health need. We believe it is important to translate existing clinical knowledge into a population-based healthcare intervention.

Keywords: male circumcision, early infant male circumcision, plastibell circumcision, task sharing, health provider, scale-up

1. Introduction

Amidst the debate on whether the benefits of circumcision outweigh risks, regardless of the reason for circumcision and irrespective of geographical, ethical and socio-economic boundaries, circumcision continues to be one of the commonest surgical procedures performed globally [1]. Since male circumcision (MC) is universal in Muslim and Jewish populations, circumcision prevalence of 99.9% was estimated, and in non-Muslim, non-Jewish states, a minimum prevalence of 0.1% was assumed to calculate the global MC prevalence of 37–39% [2]. This estimate is higher than the one given by the WHO in 2008 which was 30% [3]. The reason for the rise in MC prevalence could be attributed to the rising number of Muslims worldwide [4, 5] and to the initiation of voluntary medical male circumcision (VMMC) programmes encouraged by the WHO and the joint United Nations agency programme on HIV/AIDS—UNAIDS in sub-Saharan African countries as a preventative strategy to curb the rising incidence of HIV [2].

2. Scale of practice

2.1 Burden of circumcision

According to the *CIA World Factbook*, the annual global birth rate is estimated to be more than 134.5 million births [6]; assuming half of these to be males and using the above-mentioned global MC prevalence, 25.5 million potential circumcision procedures are required across the globe every year. Religion, culture and medical reasons are the main indications prompting families to opt for circumcision.

2.1.1 Religious considerations

An estimated 23.2% of the world's population comprise Muslims with nearly 69% of them residing in Asia and 27% in Africa [4]; 0.2% are Jews, 80% of whom live either in Israel or the USA; religious traditions in both communities staunchly advocate circumcision.

Taking Pakistan as an example of a developing Muslim country in Asia, an estimated 2.5 million male babies are born in Pakistan every year [6], almost all of whom undergo circumcision in their infancy or childhood [3]. Presently, the vast majority of circumcisions are performed by traditional circumcisers, barbers and untrained paramedical staff using unsterilized instruments and unsafe techniques with no follow-up or record of any complications; only 5–10% of boys present to qualified surgeons and physicians [7]. It would be unreasonable to rely on specialists and general practitioners to fulfill this huge unmet need for safe circumcisions, given that the estimated physician density in Pakistan is 0.978 per 1000 with only about 200 registered pediatric surgeons in the country [8]. In countries where healthcare resources are insufficient, emphasis needs to shift towards developing a public health strategy whereby appropriate non-medical personnel are trained to perform circumcisions safely, using correct technique and modern infection control practices [9].

2.1.2 Cultural requirements

For thousands of years, traditional circumcision has been practiced in African tribes of sub-Saharan region and amongst many ethnic groups around the world, including aboriginal Australasians, the Aztecs and Mayans in the Americas and in the Philippines [3]. The prime reason for circumcision in most of these groups is to emphasize and celebrate the occasion of rite of passage to manhood.

2.1.3 Medical indications

Around 80 percent of American men are circumcised, one of the highest rates in the developed world [10]. The USA is the only country in the world where newborn circumcision in male babies is highly prevalent, allegedly for health benefits [11], and an overwhelming majority gets circumcised in hospitals, soon after birth [12]. According to estimates, 80–95% of male infants were being circumcised in the USA by the 1970s [13]. The US Centers for Disease Control and Prevention (CDC) proclaimed that this trend showed a decline thereafter, possibly influenced by the pronouncements of the American Academy of Pediatrics (AAP) in 1971, deeming there are no valid medical indications for circumcision in the neonatal period [14]. The CDC, however, collects voluntary data only from participating hospitals, some of which withdrew neonatal circumcision services due to financial reasons, thereby displaying sharp decline in circumcision rates in those particular settings [11, 13]. Many hospitals chose to discontinue coding circumcisions as procedures which may have led to inaccuracy in the collected data; moreover, circumcisions performed during subsequent hospital admissions or as outpatients were not recorded. Therefore, accurate conclusions about the actual number of procedures being performed cannot be drawn. Nelson et al. reported that the incidence of newborn circumcision increased steadily between 1988 and 2000 in the USA from 48.3 to 61.1%, with the overall weighted incidence of circumcision being 54.4% [12]. Revision in the stance of AAP Task Force on Circumcision in 1989 to a more neutral position that stated 'Circumcision has potential medical benefits and advantages as well as disadvantages and risks' and that parental decisions should be based on informed consent, could be a possible factor influencing the circumcision rates. Availability of health insurance is another important factor favorably influencing the numbers of circumcisions [15]. Being the commonest surgical procedure performed in the USA, circumcision exerts a considerable impact on the health system of the country; on one hand, it usurps the medical budget by utilizing the health personnel and consumables that collectively build towards the direct cost of the procedure and its associated complications, and on the other hand, it helps to reduce any potential indirect costs by diseases that are averted as a result of benefits from the procedure.

In recent years, increasing evidence has linked male circumcision to lower rates of asymptomatic urinary tract infection (UTI) [16, 17], especially during infancy and to lower risk of transmission of sexually transmitted diseases, most notably of the HIV [18]. At the end of 2006, an estimated 39.5 million people were living with HIV, and the incidence of new cases was 4.3 million that year [19]. Three randomized controlled trials were conducted to assess the impact of MC on HIV risk [20–22]; all three studies were aborted when interim analysis showed compelling evidence that MC reduces the risk of acquiring HIV through heterosexual sex by 51–60%. This led to global attention on this procedure, thereby encouraging prophylactic circumcision in many countries with a high prevalence of HIV/AIDS [23], especially in sub-Saharan Africa. The WHO/UNAIDS recommended rapid scale-up of MC in settings where prevalence of heterosexually transmitted HIV infection is high, the levels of male circumcision are low, and populations at risk of HIV are large.

Africa has a unique burden of circumcision with many Muslim-majority countries, a high prevalence of HIV in many countries and cultural preferences in certain tribes. Somalia, a sub-Saharan African Muslim country displaying a very high birth rate and inadequate health services, has an unimpressive physician density of 0.02 per 1000. Uganda has 13.7% Muslims, with a high birth rate, physician density of 0.09 per 1000 coupled with a high burden of HIV cases. Kenya, accommodating 11.2% Muslims, with a high birth rate superimposed with a huge burden of HIV cases and a physician density of 0.2 per 1000 shows 84% of all Kenyan men are circumcised, predominantly due to cultural obligation [3].

3. Interventional strategies

Circumcisions prompted by religious, cultural or general health benefits are not an emergency. However, those required to control the spread of HIV epidemic globally are urgent, and crucial steps need to be taken to ensure their instatement. Therefore, the implementation of 'voluntary medical male circumcision' and 'early infant male circumcision' (EIMC) programmes to tackle HIV spread and high volumes of routine circumcisions, respectively, provide plausible solutions.

3.1 Voluntary medical male circumcision

3.1.1 Counseling and dissemination of correct information

First and foremost, factual information should be clearly provided to high-risk communities in general and to the men opting for circumcision and their partners in particular. MC has shown to reduce, *not eliminate*, the risk of acquiring HIV through heterosexual sex; it is not known whether MC directly reduces sexual transmission of HIV from HIV-positive men to women or if MC has a protective role in men who have sex with men (MSM). MC should be considered only as an adjuvant to therapy along with other HIV prevention measures, and it should not mislead circumcised individuals into considering high-risk sexual behaviors as inconsequential. Additionally, it should be conveyed that abstinence from sexual activity is required after circumcision for at least 6 weeks to ensure that the wound has healed completely; otherwise the circumcised men would be at a higher risk for contracting HIV from an infected partner, or if HIV-positive, then there would be a higher risk of infecting their sexual partners.

3.1.2 VMMC: a preventative strategy

The vast majority of people living with HIV belong to low- and middle-income countries, particularly in Africa. Immediate intervention proposed by the WHO/UNAIDS in 2007 for impeding HIV spread was provision and rapid scale-up of VMMC services in at least 14 vulnerable countries in Africa where HIV prevalence was high, spread was predominantly through heterosexual transmission, and MC levels were low [24]. Target was to achieve 20 million circumcisions in HIV-negative men by 2016. By the end of 2013, only 30% of the target was achieved, and a joint strategic action framework was devised by UNAIDS, the WHO and other stake-holders to review the steps in order to expedite the scale-up of VMMC to fulfill the desired goal [25]. Although the time-bound ultimate target seemed ambitious to be achieved by 2016 mainly due to large numbers of trained healthcare workers required along with a continuous flow of funds [24], all involved countries showed an increase in the pace of scale-up of VMMC programmes leading to 12 million circumcisions of adolescent boys and men by the end of 2015 [26]. This proximity to the target encouraged UNAIDS and the WHO to launch a new, more holistic framework for action—VMMC2021. This document gives newer strategic directions on VMMC for HIV prevention and envisions that 90% of males aged 10–29 years will have been circumcised by 2021, in priority settings in sub-Saharan Africa.

It should be kept in mind that VMMC is unlikely to provide public benefit in areas where HIV prevalence is low or is concentrated in specific populations such as intravenous drug users, MSM or sex workers.

3.2 Early infant male circumcision

Whereas VMMC programmes have been popularly introduced and implemented in high-risk populations, there is a comparative absence of EIMC programmes in relevant countries. To promote the safe circumcision initiative, a manual was developed by joint efforts of the WHO and JHPIEGO in 2010, which also provided the technical guidance for structuring an EIMC [27]. However, large-scale adoption of this recommendation by stakeholders is yet to be seen. For effective implementa-tion, a careful needs assessment should be conducted in advance to investigate the expected scale of requirement.

3.2.1 Muslim-majority countries

Promotion of early infant male circumcision programmes could be a simple, safe, reasonable and economical strategy in countries where burden of circumcision is high, financial constraints are present, and standard of healthcare services is low. In Muslim-majority countries like Pakistan, male circumcision is considered an essential religious practice; there is unanimous consensus that the male baby should be circumcised. Therefore, the focus needs to be on ensuring that these circumcisions are performed safely, as early as possible in life with the lowest possible risk of complications. Introduction of service delivery programmes, promoting and delivering safe, sterile early infant circumcisions at a subsidized cost or as part of the free public sector healthcare package, could provide a meaningful and long-term solution.

3.2.2 Developing countries with high-HIV prevalence

The WHO/UNAIDS and UNICEF also recommend EIMC be implemented simultaneously with scale-up of MC services as a long-term strategy for the control of HIV. Modeling studies show promising results for universal MC in sub-Saharan Africa, claiming it could significantly reduce morbidity and mortality associated with HIV over time [19]. For effective execution of EIMC services, maternal and infant health programmes need to be engaged as well.

3.2.3 Developed countries with a high circumcision burden

In countries like the USA with a high prevalence of circumcision or in other developed countries like the UK with pockets of Muslim-majority communities, the need for these procedures is high. Since medical insurance does not cover circumcision, there is risk of this procedure being restricted to affluent or insured patients, as indicated by falling circumcision rates in the USA in patients without insurance coverage [12, 15]. EIMC programmes introduced in these settings could fulfill the patient requirements as well as bring about significant cost reduction associated with the procedure.

4. Implementation and scale-up of EIMC programmes

The key aspects for successful implementation and scale-up of EIMC include training of health workers, developing programme infrastructure, ensuring supply of equipment and consumables, identifying funding and establishing robust monitoring and evaluation systems and policy development.

4.1 Training of health providers

Health providers need to be provided with theoretical knowledge about basic anatomy of the area and details of the surgical technique [1, 27, 28] and possible complications related to the procedure. This should be followed by practical demonstration of the technique. A US-based training programme employed the Gomco clamp method of circumcision [13] to train certified nurse-midwives (CNMs) in 1981, under supervision of obstetricians. In 1996, volunteer nurses in the UK were trained by consultant urologists to perform Plastibell circumcisions. A similar protocol is being followed by an EIMC programme established in Karachi, Pakistan, since 2016, in which pediatric surgeons are training OR technicians, midwives, health workers and family physicians to perform circumcisions using the Plastibell method.

These training programmes have adopted a similar approach with theoretical training followed by skills teaching, initially performing procedures under close supervision, and subsequently independently with routine monitoring of outcomes. At the end of the training period, a knowledge and skills assessment is carried out before the health providers are certified to practice. This process allows the procedure to be performed safely and efficiently in settings where large numbers of circumcisions are required.

4.1.1 Types of providers

Task sharing is a well-established approach worldwide, whereby health providers are trained to perform high volume, technically less demanding tasks, under close supervision and monitoring with a referral system in place [29]. The 'manual for early infant male circumcision under local anaesthesia' by the WHO recommends that early infant male circumcision should primarily be the task of nonphysician healthcare workers which include, but are not limited to, nurses, midwives, clinical officers, health officers and assistant medical officers. Non-specialist medical doctors can also be trained for this procedure. The competence of the providers is the single most important factor affecting the outcome of the procedure and, hence, is critical to the success of any large-scale implementation.

Non-medical, religious providers called 'mohels', trained and supervised by the Ministry of Religion and the Ministry of Health, perform circumcisions in Israel [9]. Trained and certified nurses and midwives are another pool of non-medically trained providers that commonly perform this procedure in West Africa. Medically trained providers include obstetricians, pediatricians, general practitioners, general surgeons or pediatric surgeons and urologists, who routinely undertake ritual neonatal circumcisions in hospital settings commonly in countries like the USA and the Gulf states, in addition to performing therapeutic circumcisions in countries around the world.

The selection of the provider is influenced by preference of the family, the cost of the procedure, location, accessibility, culture and socio-economic status of the parents. If adequate numbers of physicians and specialists are available to run an EIMC, this may be the preferred approach in resource-rich settings. The real challenge arises in resource-constrained settings, especially in rural areas, where families approach traditional, untrained providers since they are the only viable option due to convenience, proximity or cost dynamics [9]. In Pakistan, 90–95% of circumcisions are performed by untrained barbers, technicians, religious or traditional circumcisers [7], who remain oblivious to the associated risks and are unable to handle complications that occur far too frequently. Similarly, barbers or traditional circumcisers are the popular choice in Egypt, Turkey and Iran for this procedure [9]. Not surprisingly, these untrained and unmonitored providers pose the biggest threat, with short- and long-term sequelae being the norm.

Links between the formal and informal health sectors could help increase the safety and quality of the procedure and enhance the monitoring and evaluation aspect of the program. In Accra (the capital of Ghana), where neonatal circumcision is almost universal, good links have been established between the Public Health Service and traditional circumcisers in order to provide regular training in safe infant circumcision. Similar models should be explored in other settings.

Circumcision is a simple surgical procedure that can be safely performed by a trained person. It does not have to be done by a doctor or a specialist. All types of health providers, whether they are surgeons, nurses, technicians or traditional circumcisers [7, 27, 28, 30], have shown comparable results as long as they are adequately trained.

4.1.2 Circumcision techniques

The three common methods of neonatal or early infant circumcision include Plastibell, Mogen clamp and Gomco clamp. Providers can be trained to perform any of these techniques as all of them have comparable safety profiles [27, 31]. Adoption of a single method is recommended to ensure standardization of technique in order to facilitate the training of the providers and their monitoring by making fair comparisons based on occurrence of complications; additionally, employment of a single method enables ease of procurement for the program. Plastibell technique of circumcision is a simple method that is easily taught and can be performed safely by health providers with low complication rates [31–34]. However, the clamping devices may be safer for EIMC in regions where follow-up services to deal with complications, like retained rings, are unavailable [33].

4.2 Programme infrastructure

EIMC programmes best serve their purpose and provide maximum benefit to communities when they are integrated into existing healthcare systems such as the maternal, neonatal and child health (MNCH) programmes. For example, introduction of such programmes at birthing or vaccination centres is advised, where a stream of age-appropriate patients is already expected. Targeting these places would result in early and successful establishment of these programmes. Vertical, solitary programmes may be useful as short-term, pilot programmes or as training centres for health providers in areas where circumcision rates are high and healthcare systems are weak. Once piloted, replication and scale-up strategies should be employed to achieve sustainability.

4.2.1 Timing of circumcision–a critical factor

Circumcision can be performed at any age. Judaism proposes the eighth day of life in a healthy baby; in Islam, the time could be anywhere between birth and puberty. In some Muslim countries like Pakistan, cultural pressures influence the timing of circumcision. The ritual is ordained to be celebrated as a festive occasion with special arrangements including dinner, requiring the presence of relatives and friends, especially amongst certain ethnic groups. This exerts an unnecessary financial strain on the families who often delay the circumcision of their babies till they have enough money to organize the event, which often makes them cross the beneficial age-limit of 2 months following birth. In order to discourage this practice and to create awareness amongst masses regarding the advantages of early infant circumcision, a video was developed in the national language as a tool for information dissemination by an EIMC programme established in Karachi, Pakistan. The link to this Video 1 (with English subtitles) is available here: https://bit.ly/38be8P5.

From the medical point of view, the neonatal period offers the best opportunity for circumcision with avoidance of general anesthesia and its associated challenges; additionally, it provides all possible benefits of circumcision to the baby as early as possible in life, with better and early chances of recovery, lower cost and a lower incidence of post-procedure complications. MC should not be performed until at least 24 hours after birth to ensure the infant is stable and has had time to void, feeding has initiated, and abnormalities, if any, become apparent [27]. Therefore, for large-scale EIMC programmes, early procedures performed from the second day of birth up to 2 months, in otherwise healthy babies, are preferred [27, 35]. Since circumcision is an elective procedure, it should be deferred in case the baby is unwell, underweight, preterm or if any doubts surface during screening. Physiological jaundice is not considered a contraindication; however, if the baby is deeply jaundiced, circumcision should be deferred, and referral for appropriate work up and management should be initiated as soon as possible [35, 36]. Ethical arguments propose that circumcision should be deferred till the patient is old enough to make his own decision; however, delaying or postponing the procedure negates the protective effect of circumcision required as early in life as possible and the concomitant reduced-cost benefit due to avoidance of general anesthesia.

4.2.2 Programme prerequisites

During the 1970s in the USA when circumcision rates were at their peak, the procedure was considered so beneficial that many hospitals did not require a written consent [13]. However, in 2012, the Task Force on Circumcision (which included members of the American Academy of Pediatrics (AAP), American Academy of Family Physicians (AAFP), American College of Obstetricians and Gynecologists (ACOG) and Centers for Disease Control and Prevention) stated that 'benefits of circumcision outweigh its risks' and strong recommendations were made to obtain 'informed consent' from parents or guardians prior to the procedure [1].

While establishing neonatal male circumcision programmes, the Task Force on Circumcision and the WHO [27] also recommend vitamin K to be routinely administered to the babies before the procedure in order to help prevent post-procedure bleeding. Routine pre-procedure investigations are not advocated nor justified in large-scale EIMC programmes [35]. Circumcision is contraindicated in babies born with genital abnormalities (like epispadias, hypospadias, chordee, ambiguous genitalia, micropenis, buried penis, penoscrotal web or bilateral hydrocele), blood dyscrasias or those with a family history of bleeding disorders.

Additionally, pain relief should be provided to the infant during the procedure. For this purpose, dorsal penile nerve block or ring block could be employed; the former has the advantages of lesser number of pricks and a shorter duration of onset.

4.2.3 Post-procedure care

If trained providers perform the procedure, post-circumcision complications are generally minor and easily managed. However, they can and do occur, even in the best hands. Health providers should be equipped to handle simple post-procedure complications like minor bleeding requiring application of pressure with or without topical adrenaline or simple cutting and removal of a Plastibell ring that fails to shed spontaneously. If these complications occur in post-clinic hours, then a referral system to handle these or other common complications following circumcision ensures the success of EIMC programmes. The ongoing recruitment and training of health providers in large-scale programmes poses a constant challenge in terms of high chances of occurrence of complications by new trainees; this can be addressed by a reliable referral system to handle these when the need arises.

4.2.4 Patient follow-up and outcome documentation

Patient follow-up and outcome determination are of utmost importance in any public health intervention. In EIMC programmes, active and passive follow-up after the procedure allows documentation of post-procedure adverse events and helps assess parental satisfaction with the process. Diligent and regular review of data allows the programme team to monitor quality and safety outcomes and address any challenges that may be identified. Refresher training and modification of technique or approach may be instituted to address any issues that may arise. A helpline or open access to the clinic allows patients to call or come in with concerns that can either be adequately dealt with by the primary team or referred appropriately.

Low literacy levels, socio-economic constraints and geographical barriers are all hurdles to early recognition and reporting of complications, which if left unattended, could lead to serious adverse events following a simple procedure like neonatal circumcision [37]. Regular engagement between providers delivering health services and families in the communities, to counsel them before and after the procedure, helps build a rapport which is the basis of successful public health programmes. This bond could be utilized by the providers to probe and carry out a qualitative analysis to judge the acceptability of the programme by the community or to find ways to improve the services by getting direct input from the biggest stakeholders in this arrangement. On the other hand, the health providers could be the source of correct information and guidance for these communities regarding various aspects of health promotion. Participants of the programme usually share their experiences with others in the community; reputation, good or bad, spreads through word of mouth, either encouraging or discouraging others to opt for similar services.

4.3 Programme equipment and consumables

Timely procurement of programme equipment like circumcision sets and boards, amongst others, along with adequate stock of consumables, is vital to ensure smooth running of these programmes. The major hurdle towards scale-up of this programme into the community and especially in rural areas is the limitation of availability of central sterile services department (CSSD) for sterilization of instruments used for circumcision. Scale-up of such programmes would be facilitated by the employment of pre-packed circumcision sets, containing single-use, low-cost instruments and consumables. This approach has already been adopted by VMMC programmes [24] in Africa but is currently under consideration and trial for EIMC programmes. Large-scale implementation would allow the cost of these sets to be minimized.

4.4 Funding

Countries which require establishment of EIMC programmes should draft a budget and allocate funds accordingly. Continuity of disbursement of funds is vital for programme operations. In countries where religious circumcision is needed and those with a high requirement of circumcision due to HIV prevalence, EIMC service delivery programmes should be established with no cost or lowest possible cost to the patient. Private donors and governments should consider cost saved from avoidance of occurrence of diseases like UTI and sexually transmitted diseases like HIV. Additionally, circumcisions performed on older children are costlier because of the need of general anesthesia and hospitalization; there is also an increased risk of post-circumcision complications in older children which require medical attention and, hence, account for added expense. Lastly, the societal cost of botched circumcisions in the hands of untrained providers must be avoided under any circumstances.

4.5 Monitoring and evaluation system

Strong coordination between the programme team members is important for effective functioning of the program. Adherence to programme guidelines, regular surveillance of data and management of inventory should be ensured by the programme manager. In our experience, the use of a software application for data collection allows real-time monitoring and rapid access to data for analysis which forms a critical part of a large-scale-up implementation. This also serves as an effective monitoring tool. All complications per provider should be recorded and feedback shared with the team on a regular basis to review and revise the technique as required.

Goals and objectives of the programme should be specified when the programme is being conceptualized. Goals are achieved over for a long term (5–10 years); as an example, with effective establishment of EIMC programmes, an increased prevalence of circumcision in infants should be detected. Objectives are shown by results achieved. Additionally, parameters to study the structure, process and outcome indicators should be delineated. These should be monitored routinely to assess the progress of the program. An example of an outcome indicator is the number of post-procedure complications out of the total procedures performed.

4.6 Policy development

For scale-up of EIMC programmes, it is essential that there is a legal framework supported by policies to ensure that neonatal or early infant circumcisions are performed safely. This includes obtaining informed consent from parents or guardians prior to the procedure and, in the absence of any coercive influence, use of safe technique and sterile instruments along with reliability of trained providers. Most countries display a lacking in it but Israel is an exception [9]. According to Israeli law, circumcision of baby boys up to 6 months of age is considered a religious ritual which can be performed by religious or traditional circumcisers; beyond this age, only qualified surgeons are allowed to do so. Additionally, Israeli government is directly involved in the training of traditional providers or mohels. Formulation of a national policy on similar lines, to promote safe circumcisions in Muslim-majority countries or regions, is urgently required.

Circumcisions are being done by nurses and other health providers in VMMC programmes; however, some countries like Pakistan have not looked at task sharing as a way to address the critical shortage of healthcare professionals. A national health policy framework should be developed to facilitate and encourage task sharing [29]. This has been done successfully in maternal and child health by training nonphysician clinicians (NPCs) and traditional birth attendants (TBAs) in comprehensive emergency obstetric care [38].

While circumcision is being employed as an option to curtail the number of HIV cases, it could well be the source of spread of blood-borne infections like hepatitis or HIV, if aseptic measures are not adopted [35, 39]. Circumcisions performed by untrained traditional providers in non-clinical settings with unsterilized instruments pose the greatest threat. Therefore, awareness and training of health providers to practice a safe, sterile technique in EIMC programmes is imperative for success and scale-up. Policies should be structured to ensure sterility of equipment used for circumcision.

5. Existing models of EIMC

Table 1 shows a comparison of a few EIMC programmes of somewhat similar characteristics.

Country of origin/ study reference	Year/duration of program	No. of circumcisions	Age of babies	Type of provider	No. of providers trained	Method	Complication rate
USA/ [13]	1981–1991/10 years	1000	Newborns	Certified nurse-midwives	3	Gomco clamp	0.1%
UK/ [40]	1996–1998/2 years	168	6–14 weeks	Nurses	3	Plastibell method	18%
UK/ [28]	1996–2005/9 years	1129	6–14 weeks	Nurses	Not specified	Plastibell method	8.2%
Pakistan	From 2016 (ongoing)	3755	Up to 3 months	OR technicians, midwives, health workers, family med residents	12	Plastibell method	3%

Table 1.
Comparison of EIMC programmes.

6. Conclusion

Impact of EIMC programmes can be realized immediately in countries where religious obligation is the motivation; however, impact on HIV incidence will not be evident until at least 20 years from commencement of the programmes. Implementation followed by scale-up of EIMC programmes should be encouraged as this relieves the stress on the health system of any country requiring high volumes of circumcisions. Technicians, nurses, midwives and health workers could serve as the promising pool of task-sharers to reduce the financial and technical burden without compromising on patient safety and outcomes.

Success of these programmes depends on proper training of health providers, close monitoring of outcomes and a reliable referral system. Additionally, strict adherence to programme protocols and provision of clear instructions to families on the need for early reporting of complications are essential for best results.

Conflict of interest

The authors declare no conflict of interest.

Author details

Shazia Moosa[1] and Lubna Samad[1,2]*

1 Center for Essential Surgical and Acute Care, Indus Health Network, Pakistan

2 Department of Pediatric Surgery, The Indus Hospital, Karachi, Pakistan

*Address all correspondence to: lubna.samad@ird.global

IntechOpen

References

[1] Circumcision AAoPTFo. Male circumcision. Pediatrics. 2012;**130**(3):e756

[2] Morris BJ, Wamai RG, Henebeng EB, Tobian AA, Klausner JD, Banerjee J, et al. Estimation of country-specific and global prevalence of male circumcision. Population Health Metrics. 2016;**14**(1):4

[3] World Health Organization Report. Male Circumcision: Global Trends and Determinants of Prevalence, Safety and Acceptability. Geneva, Switzerland; 2008

[4] Kettani H, editor. 2010 world muslim population. In: Proceedings of the 8th Hawaii International Conference on Arts and Humanities. 2010

[5] Kettani H. Muslim population in europe: 1950-2020. International Journal of Environmental Science and Development. 2010;**1**(2):154

[6] Central Intelligence Agency. The World Factbook. Washington D.C; 2019

[7] Rizvi S, Naqvi S, Hussain M, Hasan A. Religious circumcision: A Muslim view. BJU International. 1999;**83**(S1):13-16

[8] '200 paediatric surgeons cater to 45pc population'. Dawn Newspaper. Pakistan. March 04, 2017. [Accessed: 26 November 2019]

[9] Joint United Nations Programme on HIV/AIDS (UNAIDS). Neonatal and Child Male Circumcision: A Global Review. Geneva, Switzerland: World Health Organization Report; 2010

[10] Rabin RC. Steep Drop Seen in circumcisions in U.S. The New York Times. New York City, United States of America; 2010

[11] Wallerstein E. Circumcision. The uniquely American medical enigma.

Urologic Clinics of North America. 1985;**12**(1):123-132

[12] Nelson CP, Dunn R, Wan J, Wei JT. The increasing incidence of newborn circumcision: Data from the nationwide inpatient sample. The Journal of Urology. 2005;**173**(3):978-981

[13] Gelbaum I. Circumcision: To educate, not indoctrinate—A mandate for certified nurse-midwives. Journal of Nurse-Midwifery. 1992;**37**(S1):97S-113S

[14] Library TCR. United States Circumcision Incidence. 2010. Available from: http://www.cirp.org/library/statistics/USA/

[15] Mansfield CJ, Hueston WJ, Rudy M. Neonatal circumcision: Associated factors and length of hospital stay. Journal of Family Practice. 1995;**41**(4):370-376

[16] Simforoosh N, Tabibi A, Khalili SAR, Soltani MH, Afjehi A, Aalami F, et al. Neonatal circumcision reduces the incidence of asymptomatic urinary tract infection: A large prospective study with long-term follow up using Plastibell. Journal of Pediatric Urology. 2012;**8**(3):320-323

[17] Morris BJ. Why circumcision is a biomedical imperative for the 21st century. BioEssays. 2007;**29**(11):1147-1158

[18] Krieger JN. Male circumcision and HIV infection risk. World Journal of Urology. 2012;**30**(1):3-13

[19] WHO. New Data on Male Circumcision and HIV Prevention: Policy and Programme Implications. Geneva: WHO; 2007

[20] Auvert B, Taljaard D, Lagarde E, Sobngwi-Tambekou J, Sitta R, Puren A. Randomized, controlled intervention trial of male circumcision

for reduction of HIV infection risk: The ANRS 1265 trial. PLoS Medicine. 2005;**2**(11):e298

[21] Bailey RC, Moses S, Parker CB, Agot K, Maclean I, Krieger JN, et al. Male circumcision for HIV prevention in young men in Kisumu, Kenya: A randomised controlled trial. The Lancet. 2007;**369**(9562):643-656

[22] Gray RH, Kigozi G, Serwadda D, Makumbi F, Watya S, Nalugoda F, et al. Male circumcision for HIV prevention in men in Rakai, Uganda: A randomised trial. The Lancet. 2007;**369**(9562):657-666

[23] Kim HH, Li PS, Goldstein M. Male circumcision: Africa and beyond? Current Opinion in Urology. 2010;**20**(6):515-519

[24] Ledikwe JH, Nyanga RO, Hagon J, Grignon JS, Mpofu M, Semo B-W. Scaling-up voluntary medical male circumcision-what have we learned. HIV AIDS. 2014;**6**:139-146

[25] WHO. UNAIDS, Joint Strategic Action Framework to Accelerate the Scale-up of Voluntary Medical Male Circumcision for HIV Prevention in Eastern and Southern Africa, 2012-2016. Geneva: WHO; 2011

[26] WHO. A Framework for Voluntary Medical Male Circumcision: Effective HIV Prevention and a Gateway to Improved Adolescent boys'& men's Health in Eastern and Southern Africa by 2021. Geneva: World Health Organization; 2016

[27] WHO. Manual for Early Infant Male Circumcision under Local Anaesthesia. Geneva: World Health Organization; 2010

[28] Palit V, Menebhi DK, Taylor I, Young M, Elmasry Y, Shah T. A unique service in UK delivering Plastibell® circumcision: Review of 9-year results.

Pediatric Surgery International. 2007;**23**(1):45-48

[29] WHO. First Global Conference on Task Shifting. Geneva: WHO; 2008

[30] Chaim JB, Livne PM, Binyamini J, Hardak B, Ben-Meir D, Mor Y, et al. Complications of circumcision in Israel: A one year multicenter survey. Israel Medical Association Journal. 2005;**7**(6):368-370

[31] Bowa K, Li MS, Mugisa B, Waters E, Linyama DM, Chi BH, et al. A controlled trial of three methods for neonatal circumcision in Lusaka, Zambia. Journal of Acquired Immune Deficiency Syndromes. 2013;**62**(1):e1

[32] Moosa FA, Khan FW, Rao MH. Comparison of complications of circumcision by'Plastibell device technique'in male neonates and infants. The Journal of the Pakistan Medical Association. 2010;**60**(8):664

[33] Plank RM, Ndubuka NO, Wirth KE, Mwambona JT, Kebaabetswe P, Bassil B, et al. A randomized trial of Mogen clamp versus Plastibell for neonatal male circumcision in Botswana. Journal of Acquired Immune Deficiency Syndromes. 2013;**62**(5):e131

[34] Bode C, Ikhisemojie S, Ademuyiwa A. Penile injuries from proximal migration of the Plastibell circumcision ring. Journal of Pediatric Urology. 2010;**6**(1):23-27

[35] Jan IA. Circumcision in babies and children with Plastibell technique: An easy procedure with minimal complications-experience of 316 cases. Pakistan Journal of Medical Sciences. 2004;**20**:175-180

[36] Eroglu E, Balci S, Ozkan H, Yorukalp O, Goksel A, Sarman G, et al. Does circumcision increase neonatal jaundice? Acta Paediatrica. 2008;**97**(9):1192-1193

[37] Samad L, Jawed F, Sajun SZ, Arshad MH, Baig-Ansari N. Barriers to accessing surgical care: A cross-sectional survey conducted at a tertiary care hospital in Karachi, Pakistan. World Journal of Surgery. 2013;**37**(10):2313-2321

[38] Gessessew A, Ab Barnabas G, Prata N, Weidert K. Task shifting and sharing in Tigray, Ethiopia, to achieve comprehensive emergency obstetric care. International Journal of Gynecology & Obstetrics. 2011;**113**(1):28-31

[39] Khan N-u-Z. Circumcision–A universal procedure with no uniform technique and practiced badly. Pakistan Journal of Medical Sciences. 2004;**20**:173-174

[40] Shah T, Raistrick J, Taylor I, Young M, Menebhi D, Stevens R. A circumcision service for religious reasons. BJU International. 1999;**83**(7):807-809

Voluntary Medical Safe Male Circumcision for HIV/AIDS Prevention in Botswana: Background, Patterns, and Determinants

Mpho Keetile

Abstract

The safe male circumcision program has been running for about 10 years now, in Botswana. This chapter uses data derived from the two Botswana AIDS Impact Surveys (BAIS III and IV) conducted in 2008 and 2013, the period before and after the implementation of the SMC program to assess the background, patterns, and correlates of safe male circumcision. Data were analyzed using multivariate logistic regression models. Overall, 785 (12.5%) and 956 (25.2%) men reported to have been circumcised in 2008 and 2013, respectively. Elderly men aged 55–64 years were more likely to have been circumcised than men aged 10–24 years (APR = 3.40, CI = 2.00–5.76 in 2008 and APR = 3.63, CI = 2.36–5.57 in 2013). Men with primary or low and secondary education and those who reside in rural villages (APR = 0.70, CI = 0.54–0.89 in 2008; APR = 0.71, CI = 0.58–0.86 in 2013) were less likely to have been circumcised compared to men who resided in cities and towns. The odds of circumcision were also significantly low among never married (APR = 0.43, CI = 0.24–0.76) and cohabiting (APR = 0.45, CI = 0.26–0.80) men than once-married men in 2008. In 2013, the odds of circumcision were significantly low among married men (APR = 0.93, CI = 0.47–1.82). Understanding the background, patterns, and correlates of safe male circumcision is essential for programming and assessment of the effectiveness of the program.

Keywords: voluntary, safe male circumcision, HIV/AIDS, prevention, Botswana

1. Background

Male circumcision is not a new practice in Africa. It has been practiced for thousands of years as a ritual and a rite of passage to manhood [1, 2]. Similarly, in Botswana, male circumcision has been practiced as far as 1875, marked by an initiation ceremony into manhood called "bogwera" [3]. During the *bogwera* ceremony, young adolescent males were taken through a month-long period of seclusion into the wilderness where they were taught survival skills, tribal laws, and customs [4]. The bogwera was not practiced by all tribes in Botswana; only the Balete and Bakgatla tribes were participating in this ceremony [5]. In 1917, the British High Commissioner to Botswana passed a law to abolish initiation ceremonies, indicating that they were unhygienic and cruel [6].

In 1985, Botswana had the first HIV/AIDS case. Ever since from that time, a series of response plans and programs have been devised to reduce HIV transmission. In the early 2000s, epidemiological studies observed a significant association between circumcision and low HIV/AIDS prevalence [7–9]. It was found that countries with high circumcision rates recorded the lowest HIV/AIDS prevalence rates, in West, East, and Southern Africa [1]. Most of the studies conducted in these regions found that circumcision reduced vulnerability to HIV [10–12]. In order to provide conclusive empirical evidence, three randomized clinical trials were conducted to assess the effects of safe male circumcision for the prevention of HIV infection through heterosexual contact in South Africa, Uganda, and Kenya [13–15]. These trials congruently showed that HIV transmission was reduced by over 60% among circumcised men.

Owing to the evidence of the protective effects of circumcision against HIV transmission, several studies were undertaken in Botswana. Initial studies assessed the acceptability of safe male circumcision (SMC) among men in Botswana [16]. Subsequently, a mathematical model was used to calculate the public health impact of large safe male circumcision for HIV prevention. It was found that male HIV prevalence reduced from 30 to 10% and female HIV prevalence was reduced from 40 to 20% [17]. In 2009 the government of Botswana through the Ministry of Health and Wellness adopted the voluntary safe male circumcision program [17]. A 5-year strategy was then developed, which aimed at reaching 80% circumcision coverage [17]. According to Dickson et al. [18], less than 20% of males in Botswana had access to male circumcision services in 2010. Although the SMC program has been running for about 10 years in Botswana, recent evidence indicates that the program has failed to achieve its intended coverage [3].

This chapter is therefore intended to provide the background and assess the patterns and correlates of safe male circumcision within the context of a high HIV/AIDS prevalence setting. The chapter starts by providing a brief background on male circumcision and the SMC program in Botswana. It goes on to assess the patterns and determinants of SMC since the introduction of the program in 2009. An understanding of the background, patterns, and correlates of safe male circumcision is essential for programming and assessment of the effectiveness of the program.

2. Theoretical framework

This chapter generally adopts a multifaceted approach that considers HIV/AIDS risk perception among circumcised men by assessing patterns of circumcision and factors associated with circumcision among men in Botswana. This is done with the assumption that circumcision can only be effective in the context where men consider its health benefits. Most public health studies have often used individual and social behavioral theories to explain why individuals are willing to undertake a certain action and why they behave the way they do [19–22]. Individual behavior models focus on the role of individual characteristics in controlling individual behavior. Thus they focus on how individuals control their behaviors and make reasoned actions that impact those decisions [23]. On the other hand, social models include social pressures, peer influences, cultural expectations, economic factors affecting resource availability, legal and political

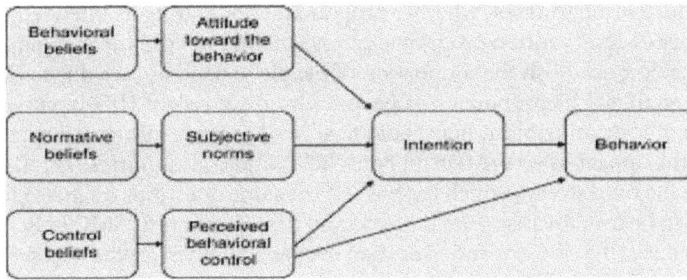

Figure 1.
Theory of reason action [25].

structures, and political and religious ideologies that restrict individual's options and the flow of information [23].

Among the various individual and social behavioral models, the theory of reasoned action (TRA) has been selected and used in this chapter to explain why men would or would not circumcise. The TRA was developed and revised numerous times by Ajzen and Fishbein [24, 25]. This theory proposes that behavioral intentions are a combined function of the attitude toward performing a particular behavior in a given situation and of the norms perceived to govern that behavior multiplied by the motivation to comply with those norms [26]. The assumption is that human beings are usually quite rational and make systematic use of the information available to them. People consider the implications of their actions before they decide to engage or not engage in a given behavior [25].

As circumcision is recommended for medical reasons (especially prevention of HIV acquisition), men who may choose circumcision must also believe that circumcision may reduce chances of HIV acquisition. This model was mainly chosen because, the constructs of this model are key in informing men's decision to accept circumcision. The assumption of TRA is that most behaviors of social bearing are under voluntary control and that a person's intention to perform or not do the behavior is the direct determinant of that action [25]. Consequently, men's intention regarding SMC is determined by personal and social influences. One personal factor is the person's evaluation of the outcome of circumcision, which can be either positive or negative.

Men who perceive that circumcision is necessary for reduction of HIV transmission may choose the procedure. Meanwhile men who believe otherwise may have negative evaluation of circumcision and may choose not to circumcise. Subjective norm is the other determinant of a person's intention which is a person's perception of the social pressures applied to perform the behavior [25]. As illustrated in **Figure 1**, an individual's intentions and behaviors are influenced by certain background factors which include individual, social, and information factors.

3. Methodology

3.1 Data

Data used in this chapter was derived from the two Botswana AIDS Impact Surveys (BAIS III and IV). BAIS III was conducted in 2008 before the implementation of SMC program, while BAIS IV was conducted in 2013 after the implementation of the SMC program. The main objectives of the BAIS were to provide information to assess whether programs are operating as intended; assess performance of intervention programs; assess whether people are changing their sexual behavior; establish the proportion of people in need of care due to HIV infection; establish the proportion of people who are at risk of HIV infection; assess the impact of the pandemic at household level; and provide information on issues related to the impact of HIV/AIDS on households and communities [27]. BAIS III and IV are the two surveys which have asked the same questions on male circumcision that can be used to assess the patterns and determinants of SMC in Botswana. A sample consisting of 6290 and 3787 men in ages 10–64 years who had successfully completed BAIS III and IV individual questionnaires, respectively, were selected and included for analyses. Respondents who did not complete the individual questionnaire were excluded from the present analysis.

3.2 Response variable

The main variable of interest used in this paper is on "circumcision status." This is based on the percentage of circumcised men between ages 10 and 64 years in the sample population. This variable is derived from self-reported responses to a question that sought to know whether the respondent was circumcised or not.

3.3 Explanatory variables

Sociodemographic variables such as age, sex, residence, education, and religion were used as control variables based on prior empirical research which has shown that conceptually these variables are associated with sexual risk behaviors [28, 29].

3.4 Statistical analysis

Analyses were conducted using SPSS version 25 program (IBM, SPSS, Chicago, IL, USA). In order to assess patterns of circumcision, adjusted prevalence ratios (APR) and their corresponding 95% confidence intervals were obtained using modified Poisson regression models. The associations between male circumcision and sociodemographic and behavioral factors were estimated for each of the surveys. In order to avoid cofounding effects between circumcision and covariates, sociodemographic variables were used as control variables. This ensured that the association between behavioral variables and circumcision becomes credible and discernible. In the adjusted analyses of sexual risk behaviors, sociodemographic characteristics were controlled for. In order to control for cluster effects, complex samples module in SPSS has been used since multistage probability sampling technique was used for both surveys.

4. Results

4.1 Patterns of safe male circumcision in Botswana (2008–2013)

Overall 785 (12.5%) and 956 (25.2%) men in the sample reported to have been circumcised in 2008 and 2013, respectively (**Figure 2**).

Table 1 shows the sociodemographic characteristics of circumcised men in Botswana (2008 and 2013). The proportion of men who were circumcised decreased with age for both surveys. For instance, in both surveys the highest proportions of circumcised men were found in ages 10–24 (25 and 28.7% for 2008 and 2013, respectively) and lowest in ages 55–64 years (8.3 and 9.8% for 2008 and 2013,

25.2

12.5

| 2008 | 2013 |

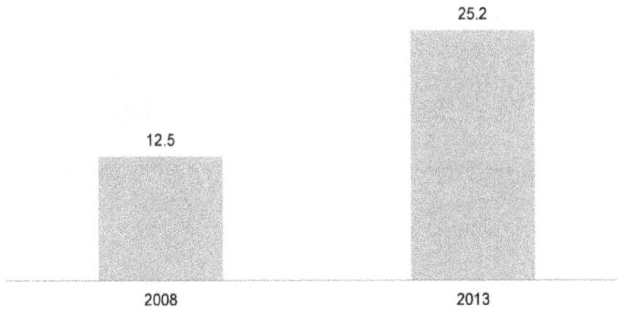

Figure 2.
Percentage of circumcised men in Botswana (2008 and 2013). Source: Analyzed from Botswana AIDS Impact Surveys III and IV (2008 and 2013).

Variables	2008 BAIS		2013 BAIS	
	Circumcised, % (n)	N	Circumcised, % (n)	N
Age				
10–24	25.0 (184)	2680	28.7 (274)	1490
25–34	31.8 (234)	1600	27.6 (264)	954
35–44	21.8 (160)	934	21.2 (203)	680
45–54	13.1 (96)	586	12.7 (121)	399
55–64	8.3 (61)	318	9.8 (94)	264
Education				
Primary/less	13.7 (78)	841	18.8 (161)	930
Secondary	53.1 (302)	2558	49.5 (423)	1688
Tertiary/higher	33.2 (189)	894	31.7 (271)	724
Residence				
Cities and towns	38.4 (282)	1739	44.1 (422)	1398
Urban villages	31.0 (228)	1901	25.9 (248)	948
Rural villages	30.6 (225)	2478	29.9 (286)	1441
Marital status				
Never married	47.8 (351)	3866	53.7 (513)	2306
Married	24.4 (179)	874	21.9 (209)	635
Cohabiting	23.4 (172)	1251	22.2 (212)	787
Once married	4.5 (33)	127	2.3 (22)	59
Religion				
Christian	64.4 (426)	3686	81.4 (778)	3089
Other non-Christian	35.6 (236)	2031	18.6 (178)	698
Total	12.5 (785)		25.2 (956)	

Table 1.
Characteristics of circumcised men aged 10–64 years in Botswana (2008 and 2013).

respectively). A high proportion of circumcised men in both surveys was found among those with secondary education in 2008 and 2013 (53.1 and 49.5%, respectively), cities and towns (38.4 and 44.1%, respectively), never married individuals (47.8 and 53.7%), and Christians (64.4 and 81.4%, respectively).

Majority of men indicated that they were circumcised later in life for both surveys (56.1% in 2008 and 52.7% in 2013). However, the proportion of men who were circumcised in later life was highest in 2008. As for the place of circumcision, a high proportion of men reported that they were circumcised in a health facility, and this was high in 2013 (78.8%) than in 2008 (69%). Under one-tenth of men (9.3% in 2008 and 7.1% in 2013) reported that they experienced some complications during circumcision. The proportion of men who expressed willingness to be circumcised in was highest in 2008 (58.6%) than in 2013 (49.5%) (**Table 2**).

4.2 Determinants of safe male circumcision in Botswana

Results in **Table 3** present the adjusted odd ratios for the association between safe male circumcision and sociodemographic factors in 2008 and 2013. Age was observed to be a significant correlate of male circumcision in both 2008 and 2013. The odds of safe male circumcision increased with age for both survey periods, with men aged 55–64 years three times (APR = 3.40, CI = 2.00–5.76 in 2008 and APR = 3.63, CI = 2.36–5.57 in 2013) more likely to have been circumcised than men aged 10–24 years. Considering education level, men with primary or less and secondary education were less likely to have been circumcised than men with tertiary or higher education level for both survey periods.

Men in rural villages were less likely to have been circumcised than men who resided in cities and towns in 2008 (APR = 0.70, CI = 0.54–0.89) and 2013 (APR = 0.71, CI = 0.58–0.86). On the other hand, there were no significant variations observed for circumcision and residing in urban villages. The odds of circumcision were significantly low among never married (APR = 0.43, CI = 0.24–0.76) and cohabiting (APR = 0.45, CI = 0.26–0.80) men than once-married men in 2008, while for married men there was no significant variation. In 2013, the odds of

Variable	2008 BAIS III		2013 BAIS IV	
	%	N	%	N
Time of circumcision?				
At birth	40.3	299	38.1	331
Later in life	56.1	416	52.7	537
Do not know	3.6	27	9.2	88
Place of circumcision?				
Health facility	69	511	78.8	753
Traditional	21.9	162	16.2	155
Do not know	9.1	68	5	48
Experienced complications?				
Yes	9.3	69	7.1	68
No	76.1	564	80.9	773
Do not know	14.6	108	12	115
Willingness to be circumcised in the next 12 months?				
Yes	58.6	3694	49.5	1270
No	41.4	2608	50.5	1295

Table 2.
Selected key safe male circumcision variables.

Variable	2008		2013	
	Adjusted PR	**95% CI**	**Adjusted PR**	**95% CI**
Age				
10–24	1.00		1.00	
25–34	1.76	(1.35–2.30)	1.36	(1.09–1.69)
35–44	2.43	(1.73–3.41)	1.76	(1.35–2.29)
45–54	2.54	(1.65–3.91)	2.41	(1.72–3.38)
55–64	3.40	(2.00–5.76)	3.63	(2.36–5.57)
Education				
Primary/less	0.32	(0.22–0.46)	0.36	(0.28–0.47)
Secondary	0.72	(0.57–0.91)	0.67	(0.55–0.82)
Tertiary/higher	1.00		1.00	
Residence				
Cities and towns	1.00		1.00	
Urban villages	0.79	(0.63–1.00)	0.90	(0.74–1.10)
Rural villages	0.70	(0.54–0.89)	0.71	(0.58–0.86)
Marital status				
Never married	0.43	(0.24–0.76)	1.10	(0.55–2.18)
Married	0.68	(0.39–1.18)	0.93	(0.47–1.82)
Cohabiting	0.45	(0.26–0.80)	1.05	(0.53–2.08)
Once married	1.00		1.00	
Religion				
Christian	0.81	(0.66–1.00)	0.95	(0.77–1.18)
Other non-Christian	1.00		1.00	

Table 3.
Adjusted prevalence ratios for the association between safe male circumcision and sociodemographic factors (2008 and 2013).

circumcision were significantly low among married (APR = 0.93, CI = 0.47–1.82) than once-married men, while no significant association was found for cohabiting and never married men. When considering religious affiliation, there was no variation on whether a man was from a Christian or any other religious background and circumcision.

5. Discussion

Due to high HIV prevalence and incidence rates, inadequacy of the response programs such as PMTCT program, BCIC programs, HIV testing and counseling, blood safety program, and STI management and control gave way to safe male circumcision program. The SMC program was seen as essential in adding to the existing strategies in preventing the spread of HIV infection [17]. The combination of research findings in South Africa, Kenya, and Uganda and the WHO/UNAIDS recommendations that male circumcision is efficacious in reducing HIV infection prompted the government of Botswana to scale up this component of HIV prevention and develop national policies, strategies, and implementation plans. Although

Botswana is not a traditionally circumcising society, evidence from this study indicates that male circumcision is highly acceptable in Botswana, corroborating the initial evidence [3, 5].

Majority of men who participated in the 2008 and 2013 surveys indicated that they were circumcised later in life and that they were circumcised in a health facility. A relatively low proportion of men reported that they experienced some complications during the procedure. This corroborates findings from other studies which show that when circumcision is done within hygienic clinical settings, there are minor chances of complications [1]. Common complications associated with circumcision in such settings include excessive loss of foreskin, skin bridges, amputation of the glans penis, and buried penis.

Evidence from this chapter indicates that between 2008 and 2013, the period before and after the implementation of the safe male circumcision program, the proportion of men who circumcised doubled. Although the program has not met its target [5], substantial gains have been made in getting high numbers of men to undergo circumcision. The scale-up of safe male circumcision program has benefited immensely from external funding which has supported biomedical marketing in the media including, billboard, radio, and TV advertising. Moreover, a renowned afro-pop artist was contracted as the campaign ambassador during the program in order to attract more men [5]. Additionally, specialized clinics have been set up in selected areas in addition to general public health facilities where SMC is conducted in hygienic, clinical conditions by medical practitioners [5].

On the other hand, the proportion of men who expressed willingness to undergo safe male circumcision had declined by about 10% in 2013. A plausible explanation for this decline is linked to several reasons. First, a review study on the SMC program by Katisi et al. [5] indicates that during the implementation of the program, cultural taboos such as the breaching of secrecy of the circumcision act by inclusion of women in performing circumcision procedure were introduced. Second, there are views that the traditional leadership has been left during the implementation of the program [3]. Lastly, elements of the minimum package for SMC that include counseling and voluntary HIV testing were repeatedly mentioned as other barriers that blocked men from circumcising [5]. HIV testing, in particular, seems to scare men away even if they would opt for circumcision.

Age was a significant predictor of male circumcision. For example, circumcision was found to increase with age, with highest proportions of circumcised men found in ages 55–64 years and lowest in ages 10–24 years. Similar observations were made in Uganda, where it was found that more than half of elderly men indicated that they have been circumcised compared to two-fifths of youth [30]. Although circumcision levels are lowest among young adolescents in Botswana, a study by Lane et al. [31] has shown that at the country level, deliberately prioritizing young adolescents is likely to achieve national coverage targets more quickly and cost-effectively than continuing to focus on older, harder-to-reach men. In Botswana, prioritization of younger men is critical to VMMC sustainability. As a result there is the school-going children circumcision initiative, whereby young boys are targeted to undergo circumcision through parental involvement. In this approach young boys consent to undergo circumcision through the involvement of parents. However, the decision to circumcise or not to circumcise lies with the children.

Considering education level, men with primary or less and secondary education were less likely to have been circumcised than men with tertiary or higher education level for both survey periods. This corroborates findings from other studies that men with high education and socioeconomic status have the propensity to undergo safe male circumcision compared to men with low education and poor socioeconomic status [32–34]. Educational attainment predisposes individuals to appreciate health programs better [35]. This is because men who have high education have better perception of the risk of HIV infection than men with low education. Consequently, there is need for more education and information for men with low education to take part in circumcision.

Men in rural villages were less likely to have been circumcised than men who resided in cities and towns in 2008. A plausible explanation for this scenario is that in 2008, the safe male program was not yet rolled out in the country. Moreover, men in rural areas are prone to lack of access to information and education. The odds of circumcision were significantly low among never married and cohabiting men than once-married men in 2008. This corroborates findings of a study by Mangombe and Kalule-Sabiti [36] which also found that in Zimbabwe never married and cohabiting men were less likely to circumcise. The main reason being that this cohort of men assumes that they at low risk of HIV infection. Meanwhile, other studies show the contrary that married men are at risk of infection compared to never married and cohabiting men [37].

In 2013, the odds of circumcision were significantly low among married than once-married men. Low prevalence of circumcision among married men can also be attributed to low risk of infection, especially where marital fidelity is practiced. There was no variation on whether a man was from a Christian or any other religious background and circumcision. Findings of the association between religion and circumcision are at best mixed. In some contexts, religion is a key predictor of circumcision among men [38], while in other contexts, as is the case in Botswana, it is not [39].

6. Conclusion

Safe male circumcision is as an effective additional strategy for HIV prevention. The medical benefits of SMC outweigh the risks. Age, education, residence, and marital status are significant determinants of male circumcision in Botswana. Consequently, more efforts should be geared toward educating men, especially those residing in rural areas and those in cohabiting relationships about the benefits of circumcision. Moreover, women need to be involved in understanding the benefits of male circumcision to ensure effectiveness of the SMC program.

Author details

Mpho Keetile
Department of Population Studies, University of Botswana, Gaborone, Botswana

*Address all correspondence to: mphokeet@yahoo.com

IntechOpen

References

[1] Lawal TA, Olapade-Olaopa EO. Circumcision and its effects in Africa. Translational Andrology and Urology. 2017;**6**(2):149-157. DOI: 10.21037/tau.2016.12.02

[2] Sovran S. Understanding culture and HIV/AIDS in sub-Saharan Africa. SAHARA-J: Journal of Social Aspects of HIV/AIDS Research Alliance. 2013;**10**(1):32-41. DOI: 10.1080/17290376.2013.807071

[3] Sabone M, Magowe M, Busang L, Moalosi J, Binagwa B, Mwambona J. Impediments for the uptake of the BotswanaGovernment'smalecircumcision initiative for HIV prevention. The Scientific World Journal. 2013:1-7. DOI: 10.1155/2013/38750

[4] Katide G. Female morality as entrenched in Botswana traditional teachings in initiation schools [master of ARTs degree dissertation]. 2017. Available from: https://core.ac.uk/download/pdf/95521641.pdf

[5] Katisi M, Daniel M. Safe male circumcision in Botswana: Tension between traditional practices and biomedical marketing. Global Public Health. 2015;**10**(5-6):739-756. DOI: 10.1080/17441692.2015.1028424

[6] Ministry of Health. Safe Male Circumcision- additional strategy for HIV prevention-A National Strategy. Gaborone: Government Printers; 2008

[7] Weiss HA, Halperin D, Bailey RC, Hayes RJ, Schmid G, Hankins CA. Male circumcision for HIV prevention: From evidence to action? AIDS. 2008;**22**:567-574

[8] Gray RH, Kigozi G, Serwadda D, Makumbi F, Nalugoda F, Watya S, et al. The effects of male circumcision on female partners' genital tract symptoms and vaginal infections in a randomized trial in Rakai, Uganda. The American Journal of Obstetrics and Gynecology. 2009;**200**(42):e41-e47

[9] Weiss HA, Dickson KE, Agot K, Hankins CA. Male circumcision for HIV prevention: Current research and programmatic issues. AIDS (London, England). 2010;**24** Suppl 4(04):S61-S69. DOI: 10.1097/01.aids.0000390708.66136.f4

[10] Halperin DT, Bailey RC. Male circumcision and HIV infection: 10 years and counting. Lancet. 2000;**354**(9192):1813-1815

[11] Weiss HA, Quigley MA, Hayes RJ. Male circumcision and risk of HIV infection in sub-Saharan Africa: A systematic review and meta-analysis. AIDS. 2000;**14**(15):2361-2370

[12] Moses S. Male circumcision: A new approach to reducing HIV transmission. CMAJ: Canadian Medical Association Journal. 2009;**181**(8):E134-E135. DOI: 10.1503/cmaj.090809

[13] Auvert B, Taljaard D, Lagarde E, Sobngwi-Tambekou J, Sitta R, et al. Correction: Randomized, controlled intervention trial of male circumcision for reduction of HIV infection risk: The ANRS 1265 trial. PLoS Medicine. 2006;**3**(5):e226. DOI: 10.1371/journal.pmed.0030226

[14] Bailey RC, Moses S, Parker CB, Agot K, Maclean I, Krieger JN, et al. Male circumcision for HIV prevention in young men in Kisumu, Kenya: A randomised controlled trial. Lancet. 2007;**369**(9562):643-656

[15] Gray RH, Li X, Kigozi G, et al. The impact of male circumcision on HIV incidence and cost per infection prevented: A stochastic simulation

model from Rakai, Uganda. AIDS. 2007;**21**(7):845-850

[16] Kebaabetswe P, Lockman S, Mogwe S, Mandevu R, Thior I, Essex M, et al. Male circumcision: An acceptable strategy for HIV prevention in Botswana. Sexually Transmitted Infections. 2003;**79**(3):214-219. DOI: 10.1136/sti.79.3.214

[17] Ministry of Health. Safe Male Circumcision-Additional Strategy for HIV Prevention. Gaborone, Botswana: Government Printers; 2011

[18] Dickson KE, Tran NT, Samuelson JL, Njeuhmeli E, Reed J, et al. Voluntary medical male circumcision: A framework analysis of policy and program implementation in eastern and southern Africa. PLoS Medicine. 2011;**8**(11):e1001133. DOI: 10.1371/journal.pmed.100113

[19] Bandura A. A social cognitive theory of personality. In: Pervin L, John O, editors. Handbook of Personality. 2nd ed. New York: Guilford Publications; 1999. pp. 154-196

[20] Prager K. Understanding Behaviour Change; How to Apply Theories of Behaviour Change to SEWeb and Related Public Engagement Activities. 2012. Available from: https://www.environment.gov.scot/media/1408/understanding-behaviour-change.pdf

[21] Hardcastle SJ, Hancox J, Hattar A, Maxwell-Smith C, Thøgersen-Ntoumani C, Hagger MS. Motivating the unmotivated: How can health behavior be changed in those unwilling to change? Frontiers in Psychology. 2015;**6**:835. DOI: 10.3389/fpsyg.2015.00835

[22] Davis R, Campbell R, Hildon Z, Hobbs L, Michie S. Theories of behaviour and behaviour change across the social and behavioural

sciences: A scoping review. Health Psychology Review. 2015;**9**(3):323-344. DOI: 10.1080/17437199.2014.941722

[23] Smith DJ. Imagining HIV/AIDS: Morality and perceptions of personal risk in Nigeria. Medical Anthropology. 2003;**22**(4):343-372

[24] Ajzen I, Fishbein M. The influence of attitudes on behavior. In: Albarracín D, Johnson BT, Zanna MP, editors. The Handbook of Attitudes. Mahwah, New Jersey: Lawrence Erlbaum Associates; 2005. pp. 173-222

[25] Ajzen I, Fishbein M. Understanding Attitudes and Predicting Social Behavior. Englewood Cliffs, NJ: Prentice-Hall; 1980

[26] Ajzen I. From intention to actions: A theory of planned behavior. In: Kuhl J, Bechmann J, editors. Action Control: From Cognitions to Behavior. New York: Springer-Verlag; 1985. pp. 11-39

[27] Statistics Botswana. Botswana AIDS Impact Survey III Report. Gaborone: Government Printers; 2008

[28] Baral S, Carmen HL, Grosso A, Wirtz AL, Beyrer C. Modified social ecological model: A tool to guide the assessment of the risks and risk contexts of HIV epidemics. BMC Public Health. 2013;**13**:482. Available from: http://www.biomedcentral.com/1471-2458/13/482

[29] Reisner SL, Poteat T, Keatley J, Cabral M, Mothopeng T, Dunham E, et al. Global health burden and needs of transgender populations: A review. Lancet. 2016;**388**(10042):412-436. DOI: 10.1016/S0140-6736(16)00684-X

[30] Wilcken A, Miiro-Nakayima F, Hizaamu RNB, Keil T, Balaba-Byans D. Male circumcision for HIV prevention—A cross-sectional study on awareness among young people

and adults in rural Uganda. BMC Public Health. 2010;**10**:209. Available from: http://www.biomedcentral.com/1471-2458/10/209

[31] Lane C, Bailey RC, Luo C, Parks N. Adolescent male circumcision for HIV prevention in high priority countries: Opportunities for improvement. Clinical Infectious Diseases. 2018;**66**(suppl_3):S161-S165. DOI: 10.1093/cid/cix950

[32] Auvert B, Taljaard D, Lagarde E, Sobngwi-Tambekou J, Sitta R, Puren A. Randomized, controlled intervention trial of male circumcision for reduction of HIV infection risk: The ANRS 1265 trial. PLoS Medicine. 2005;**2**(11):e298

[33] Andersson N, Cockcroft A. Male circumcision, attitudes to HIV prevention and HIV status: A cross-sectional study in Botswana, Namibia and Swaziland. AIDS Care. 2012;**24**:301-309. DOI: 10.1080/09540121.2011.608793

[34] Bridges JFP, Selck FW, Gray GE, McIntyre JA, Martinson NA. Condom avoidance and determinants of demand for male circumcision in Johannesburg, South Africa. Health Policy and Planning. 2011;**26**:298-306. DOI: 10.1093/heapol/czq064

[35] McGill N. Education attainment linked to health throughout lifespan: Exploring social determinants of health. Nations Health. 2016;**46**:1-9

[36] Mangombe K, Kalule-Sabiti I. Knowledge about male circumcision and perception of risk for HIV among youth in Harare, Zimbabwe. Southern African Journal of HIV Medicine. 2019;**20**(1):855. DOI: 10.4102/sajhivmed.v20i1.855

[37] Brown SL, Manning WD, Payne KK. Relationship quality among cohabiting versus married couples. Journal of Family Issues. 2017;**38**(12):1730-1753. DOI: 10.1177/0192513X15622236

[38] Tram KH, Bertrand JT. Correlates of male circumcision in eastern and southern African countries: Establishing a baseline prior to VMMC scale-up. PLoS One. 2014;**9**(6):e100775. DOI: 10.1371/journal.pone.0100775

[39] Ganczak M, Korzeń M, Olszewski M. Attitudes, beliefs and predictors of male circumcision promotion among medical university students in a traditionally non-circumcising region. International Journal of Environmental Research and Public Health. 2017;**14**(10):1097. DOI: 10.3390/ijerph14101097

Section 2

Complications of Circumcision

Chapter 4

Rare Yet Devastating Complications of Circumcision

Reem Aldamanhori

Abstract

Circumcision is by far the most common procedure done in hospitals of Muslim countries. Many research data have proven its benefits in protecting against numerous sexually transmitted diseases, urinary tract infections, and penile cancer in the patients and cervical cancer in partners. The procedure is quite safe, with a low overall complication rate. Most of the adverse events of circumcision are minor and can be managed conservatively. In some areas where circumcision is performed by an inexperienced individual, or are done in a non-sterile environment, or using the wrong equipment, complications requiring expert intervention are seen. Devastating results range from simple self-limiting swelling and superficial infection to the dreadful amputation to the glans or the whole phallus, necessitating an expert in reconstruction. Circumcision is a simple surgical procedure with minimal adverse events when done by competent trained medical personnel, in a well-controlled sterile environment, using the appropriate equipment.

Keywords: complications, circumcision

1. Introduction

Circumcision has been around for centuries. It is done as a routine for all newborn infant males in Muslim countries, reaching almost 100% (if no contraindications), in hospitals in Saudi Arabia. Circumcision continues to be done for a variety of religious, cultural, and medical reasons. The overall prevalence of circumcision in the United States is estimated to be about 80% for males, with most of these procedures performed in newborns [1].

A recent meta-analysis included 140 journal articles that came to the same conclusion; early infant male circumcision has immediate and lifelong benefits. It was shown to protect against urinary tract infections, phimosis, inflammatory skin conditions, candidiasis, various sexually transmitted diseases (STDs) in both sexes, genital ulcers, and penile, prostate and cervical cancer [2]. Adverse events of circumcisions are rare. The low risk in comparison to the benefit demonstrates that benefits of male circumcision surpass its risk.

Adverse events of circumcision have been difficult to measure accurately. The largest studies on measuring complication rate are mostly retrospective, and their data have generally not taken into account standardizing the variables. The timing of the procedure, the technique, the person performing the procedure, the setting, the equipment used can all change the percentage of overall complications significantly. Male circumcision has a low incidence of adverse events overall, especially if the procedure was performed during the first year of life [3]. The risk is further decreased and might be prevented, with careful consideration of the penile anatomy and the correct use of surgical equipment by trained clinicians in sterile environments. Most of the adverse events of circumcision are mild and are easily treatable. Nevertheless, severe complications might occur, demanding expert reconstruction, and might have a lifelong sequel. Here we discuss some of those adverse events.

2. Risk factors for complications

Routine circumcision is conventionally seen as a very low-risk surgical procedure, though every surgical procedure has inherent risks. Complication rates, although infrequent, may be influenced by several factors, including the patient's age, the patient's weight, and the experience of the health care personnel in performing the procedure.

2.1 Age of the patient

The rate of procedure-related complications during and after circumcision is low overall, especially if the procedure was performed during the first year of life. However, this low risk rises 10-fold to 20-fold when performed after infancy [3]. In a recent study, where 1000 children were circumcised using Plastibell, complications such as bleeding, hematoma, and swelling of the prepuce were higher in infants than neonates [4]. The study concluded that circumcision has less adverse events if done in the 1st year of life, the younger the age, the better the prognosis [4]. Another study also showed that circumcision in the newborn period was harmless with 0% complications. However, when its performed in older infants (older than 3 months) postoperative complications such as bleeding requiring intervention has risen to 30% [5]. Another study concluded that there were substantial statistical differences in circumcision revision rates between children older than 30 days and those less than 30 days of age [6]. These articles have proven that increasing age increases the chances of developing complications related to circumcision.

In contrast to that, an article has studied the complications of circumcision in premature neonates. The rate of complications of circumcision was evaluated for three different groups, new-born circumcision at a well-baby nursery, neonatal intensive care units, and special care nursery. Babies in the neonatal intensive care units and the special care nursery had a higher probability of developing circumcision-related complications compared with those in the well-baby nursery [7]. Overall, since neonatal circumcision is an elective procedure, there is no urgency in performing it if the patient is premature, has a fever or respiratory distress, but is preferred to is delay the procedure until the patient is stable.

2.2 Weight of the patient

Although circumcision is an apparently harmless procedure, the weight of the patient undergoing circumcision may affect the complication rate. An investigation of neonatal circumcision revealed that patients weighing >5.1 kg might be at higher risk of bleeding and long-term complications [8]. Physically, the higher the patient's weight, the probably thicker groin fat pad he will have. Therefore, it is explained that patients with higher weight have a higher risk of developing penile adhesions and buried penis [9]. While increased weight is not a contraindication to circumcision, it should be well-thought-out to advise parents about possible difficulties that may arise when a patient's weight is increased. Emphasis on genital hygiene is essential in patients with increased weight to help in avoiding complications.

2.3 Practitioner experience

Inadequate training of clinicians contributes to complications, as practitioners without formal training may not recognize congenital malformations might be contraindications to performing circumcisions. Patients with these abnormalities should be referred to a pediatric urologist to aid in the prevention of unsatisfactory results and complications [10]. In some rural areas were ritual circumcision is performed by the local barber or a senior family member, distressing complications up to the extent of penile amputation have been described. Many cases of glans and urethral injury have been observed. Amputation of the whole shaft of the penis after traditional ritual circumcision performed by a family member or unexperienced individual have been reported necessitating reconstructive expert in reimplantation. Untrained individuals who perform circumcisions are to be held responsible for the complications that arise and need to be stopped [11].

3. Complications related to anesthesia

Circumcision is one of the most popular surgical procedures around the world. Inadequate pain relief when performing this procedure in neonates may have long-standing psychological and physical implications. Insufficient pain control and submitting the patient to grave pain during the neonatal period, has proven to produce prolonged hypersensitivity to painful stimuli [12]. It was also proven that as adults, patients who have had painful neonatal surgery might require more opioid analgesia in comparison to patients with no previous neonatal surgery [12]. Even after the patient's initial tissue injury has healed, he may still experience pain extending beyond this period. This further highlights the importance of pain management in this tender young age.

Various types of anesthesia have been used to decrease painful stimuli during circumcision, decrease intraoperative patient movement, avoid intraoperative complications, and relieve postoperative pain. The different types of analgesia and anesthetic approaches that have been implemented in circumcision procedures have different efficacies. Some use topical analgesia such as lidocaine; others prefer nerve block. A recent meta-analysis has concluded that the dorsal penile nerve block was far more effective in pain control than a mixture of local anesthetics in infants during circumcision [13]. Local analgesics, though they may have fewer complications, are unpredictable. The effect local anesthetics have is directly dependent on the degree of absorption. The degree of absorption cannot be foretold as it is subjected to many factors such as skin thickness and amount of ointment applied. Another noteworthy issue is that local anesthetic creams need time to start its pain controlling properties (an average of an hour), while nerve blocks work immediately.

Local analgesia, due to the fact that they are topical, has much fewer self-limiting complications in comparison to the more invasive nerve block. While infrequent, burning, or stinging at the administration site, allergic reaction to the local anesthetic, skin discoloration, skin swelling, and neuritis might occur [14]. On the other hand, a dorsal penile nerve block is more invasive; the procedure of nerve block is itself painful. It also has a more significant risk of forming perineural hematomas.

Nerve injuries might occur secondary to intraneural injection. An allergic reaction might happen in the form of Urticaria or anaphylaxis, with the worst outcome being systemic anesthetic toxicity when accidentally injecting the local anesthetic in the systemic circulation [13].

4. Complications related to technique

The technique of circumcision is described in other chapters. Mainly, there are three devices for neonatal circumcision: the Gomco clamp, the Plastibell device, and the Mogen clamp. Additional tools are either modifications or are based on the main principles of these three devices.

4.1 Device used

Several techniques and devices have been described in the practice of circumcision. There was no statistically significant difference when comparing complications between the different methods performed. In one study, preputial stenosis was most frequently found in the traditional circumcision, while bleeding was more prevalent when using a Plastibell device [15]. A different controlled trial compared adverse events rate for circumcision using the three devices (the Gomco clamp, the Mogen clamp, and the Plastibell device) and showed that adverse events rate did not differ by the method [16].

4.2 Sutures

Different circumcision techniques differ in need to use sutures to close wounds and control bleeding. However, in some cases suturing of wound edges is inevitable. Suturing and the presence of a foreign body may result in wound infection, granulation tissue formation, stitch sinuses, foreign body reactions, and scarring. A study has shown that bleeding; excessive swelling, infection, and wound dehiscence are more commonly seen in sutured versus sutureless circumcisions [17]. The use of sutureless circumcision is an excellent alternative to the standard technique. It results in faster operative times and is a less expensive surgical option [18].

4.3 Cautery

Post-circumcision bleeding is probably the most disturbing early complication. Unfortunately, hemostatic techniques such as electrocautery are the first line of treatment, with no appreciation of their potential upsetting consequences. There is a lot of controversy in the use of thermocautery in circumcision routinely. Some studies report better cosmetic results and lower complication rates with the use of thermocautery devices. They give strict rules on the extent of cautery, the temperatures, and currents used, the type of blade, and technique of cautery [19].

On the other hand, numerous studies have reported the devastating complications following extensive cauterization. One case even reported a total loss of the whole phallus post-circumcision with the use of monopolar electrocautery. The patient had a total loss of the penis and required complete phallic reconstruction using flaps [20]. Although diathermy may seem like a necessity to control bleeding when performing circumcision, extensive use can lead to distressing outcomes [21]. Salvage surgery was carried out on five cases of post-circumcision using electrocautery. One of these infants presented to the emergency department with septic shock and multiorgan dysfunction secondary to infective gangrene of whole external genitalia [22].

5. Medical complications

5.1 Bleeding

Bleeding is the most frequent complication following circumcision [23]. To avoid excessive bleeding and the need to reoperation simple history taking is mandatory. Patients with bleeding diathesis and history of coagulopathies are not candidates for simple circumcision. Those patients need pediatric consultations and special consideration during the procedure.

The most common direct obstacle met during an elective neonatal circumcision was bleeding. It almost always requires only pressure or topical thrombin to achieve hemostasis [24]. There is no statistical difference in the rate of bleeding with different techniques used for circumcision. One study has compared the results of Plastibell clamp vs. classic dissection circumcision, and both were found to have a similar occurrence of immediate complications such as bleeding [25]. Another study has shown that a worn out, and overused Gomco clamp has less of a vessel crushing effect, hence more bleeding [26]. Another study has found that bleeding was more prevalent when using a Plastibell device [15].

Bleeding after circumcision either occurs from the frenular artery or the skin edges at the site of the incision. Caution is to be taken to avoid the frenular artery or carefully coagulate the frenulum to prevent delayed bleeding. It was formerly mentioned, that with age, the rate of postoperative complications, especially bleeding, have risen to 30% [5]. It was thought that the size and diameter of the vessels in the prepuce have increased with age hence the increased incidence of post-circumcision bleeding.

Bleeding after circumcision is generally easy to prevent, and if occurred can be stopped without difficulty. It is usually a minor event that rarely requires reoperation and intervention. A simple compression dressing is adequate, occasionally local administration of epinephrine and lidocaine might help aid in hemostasis [26]. The use of sutures or electrocautery is sometimes inevitable; caution is advised not to use excessive suturing material or electrocautery as that might lead to other complications. Rarely, the patient might need a transfusion or intravenous administration of clotting factors if bleeding diathesis were not previously discovered on the routine preoperative investigation [26].

5.2 Infection

Skin is a natural barrier against infection. It is expected that any breach of the skin surface may lead to infection. The presence of the penis in a wet environment (the diaper), and the proximity to stool contamination makes it a more susceptible place to infection. In spite of some precautions to avoid infections, a disruption in the skin surface may bring about infection. A study compared patients who received prophylactic antibiotics before circumcision with those who did not receive prophylaxis. Wound infection rates after circumcision with the use of prophylactic antibiotics was equal to the rate of wound infection after circumcision without the use of antibiotics [27]. Therefore, it was proven that prophylactic antibiotics did not protect against post-circumcision wound infection.

Occasionally circumcision site wound infection might occur. The rate of infection has differed from publication to the other. A systemic review has shown that the incidence of moderate to severe wound infections following circumcision depends on the practitioner and the equipment sterility [23]. It is generally minor and is demonstrated by mild swelling, erythema, redness, with signs of local inflammatory changes. It mostly resolves spontaneously with conservative measures and the emphasis on hygiene, or the simple use of topical antibiotics when necessary.

Most post-circumcision infections are self-limiting and can be treated conservatively. However, severe infection with puss formation and occasionally systemic infection might ensue. It is suspected when the patient presents with systemic symptoms such as fever, irritability, lethargy, or poor feeding. In this case, the patient needs admission, intravenous antibiotics, and wound debridement. Although infrequent, systemic post-circumcision wound infections represent a significant clinical problem. Post-circumcision infection has been reported to cause severe necrotizing fasciitis [28]. Infection of the surgical wound after the circumcision was reported to cause meningitis in the 1970s, that is not seen in the modern era of sterilization and antibiotics [29]. Post-circumcision Infectious complications must be reduced; it is feasible when done by trained and competent practitioners performing the procedure using sterile techniques [30].

6. Surgical complications

6.1 Meatal stenosis

Circumcision is the primary procedure done in the Muslim world. Meatal stenosis is one of the surgical complications that are not uncommon. It is reported that the incidence of meatal stenosis is rare in uncircumcised boys, and it is 10–26 times more in circumcised boys [31]. Being increasingly common, a careful meatal examination is indicated in any circumcised male with urinary symptoms [32]. The stenosed meatus is a meatus that has changed in its shape and width to a narrow circle from the previously normal slit-like meatus. This change is due to a circular scar formation. However, not all circular meatus are considered stenosed. There are accepted differences in meatal shape and width.

The development of the circular scar at the meatus causing meatal stenosis has been attributed to the ischemia of the meatus, with dividing the frenulum and using extensive cauterization [33]. In one study, 2307 children undergoing circumcision using Plastibell were split into two groups. One group where the frenulum was kept intact, and the other group where frenular hemostasis was performed in all cases by thermal cautery. Neonatal Plastibell circumcision with intact frenulum technique decreased the rate of meatal stenosis significantly in comparison to those who underwent circumcision with thermal cautery of the frenular artery [34].

Meatal stenosis is a frequent complication of circumcision. Meatal stenosis might be asymptomatic and does not necessitate surgical correction. Once the boy is toilet trained, symptoms may arise. Symptoms usually present as a thin stream that jets further away than usual. The stream might deflect upwards, and take longer than expected to empty the bladder completely. Urinary tract infection, urinary retention, and even renal failure might manifest if the diagnosis is not prompt. Surgical intervention with a dorsal slit meatotomy is the definitive treatment, with low rates of restenosis and need for reoperation [35]. The means of assessment following surgery are evaluated by the clinical improvement of symptoms and a better uroflowmetry after meatotomy compared to the preoperative uroflowmetry result [36].

6.2 Skin bridges

The skin is an organ that heals in miraculous ways. It has been shown that when there are two adjacent wounded edges of skin, or when there is skin infection between two surfaces, the skin might heal with adhesions. During circumcision, the foreskin is separated from the glans and then excised. This leaves the glans with superficial abrasions that consequently adhere to the circumcision wound, and skin bridges form. Penile skin bridges are adhesion between injuries or wounds in the glans and the penile shaft usually after circumcision. In uncircumcised men skin, bridges occur when there is no cleaning of the build-up of smegma underneath the foreskin. This leads to infection and the subsequent healing with skin bridges forming from the foreskin to the glans.

Adhesion of the skin of the penis, at the site of the circumcision incision, to the bare glans beyond the corona creates a skin bridge. It is an established complication of newborn circumcision. Skin bridges can vary from simple, transparent, flimsy, early forming skin bridge to a sizeable wide strip of skin bridge that might extend to replace the whole glans skin creating a circumferential bridge that produces a picture of a buried penis [37]. The resulting bridge of skin is cosmetically unacceptable, it may cause tethering with erections that might be painful or traumatic with penetration, it may cause penile torsion, or it could trap smegma causing recurrent inflammation or infection.

A simple pressure on the suprapubic fat pad in the clinic after circumcision follow-up is sufficient to separate the fragile transparent skin bridge. Careful dressing of this area until complete healing of the raw surfaces is essential to prevent a recurrence. More well-defined skin bridges might require reoperation with excision of the skin bridge [38]. Reconstruction of these adhesions includes separation of the skin bridge from the glans, excision of all abnormal skin, and meticulous dressing

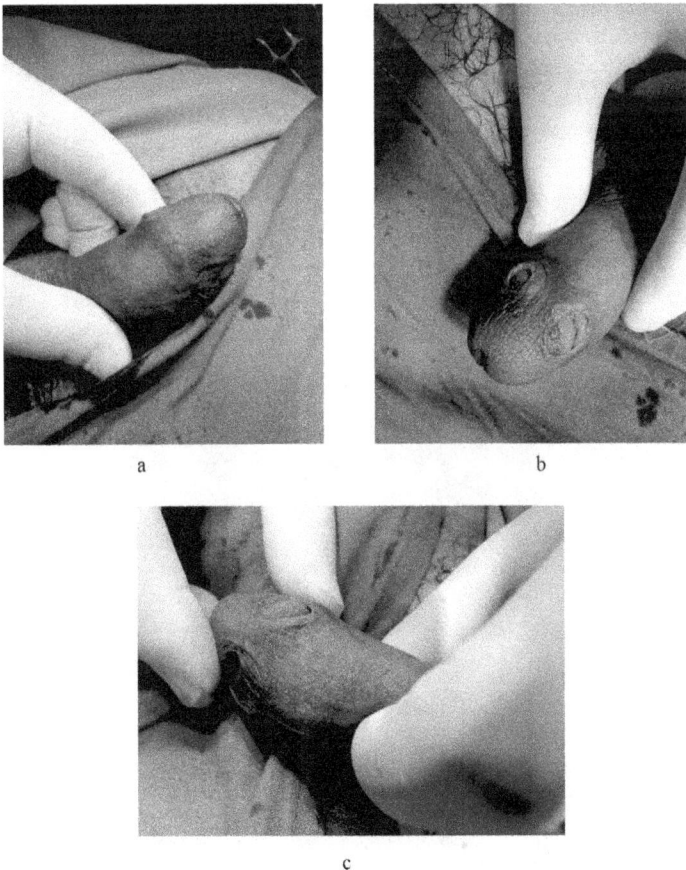

Figure 1.
(a-c) Large skin bridges covering a large surface area of the glans epithelium.

of the raw surface to prevent a recurrence. Glans epithelium subsequently heals, bringing back the typical appearance of a glans and coronal sulcus [37].

On the other hand, circumferential skin bridges might be extraordinarily disfiguring and tricky to repair. It is a challenge to divide the wide bridges from the glans without causing scarring of the glans epithelium. When the bridge is replacing a large surface area of the glans epithelium beyond the bridge, it is not merely corrected by simple bridge lysis (**Figure 1a–c**). Raw glans and an unappealing appearance of the glans might result from the correction of these types of penile skin bridges (**Figure 2**). This might need skin grafts or flaps and an expert in reconstruction [39].

In a study where a total of 277 patients were circumcised, of those patients, 26 patients experienced long-term complications, the majority being penile adhesions [8]. Buried penis, penile adhesions, and penile skin bridges are complications after circumcision that seems to occur more frequently in overweight children [9]. It was also reported that 63% of patients presenting for circumcision revision were found to have prominent suprapubic fat pads [40]. In one study where circumcised children were randomly divided into two groups depending on the method of circumcision Plastibell versus circumcision with dissection, late complications, especially adhesions, were higher in the group circumcised with dissection [25]. These limitations should be well-thought-out before new-born circumcision when counseling guardians before circumcision. Early recognition of neonatal obesity might indicate the necessity for meticulous genital hygiene to try to prevent post-circumcision complications such as skin bridges. Cautious circumcision technique, avoiding any glans injury, and proper dressing at the time of circumcision are simple actions that can prevent adherence of the distal perpetual skin flap to the glans penis [39].

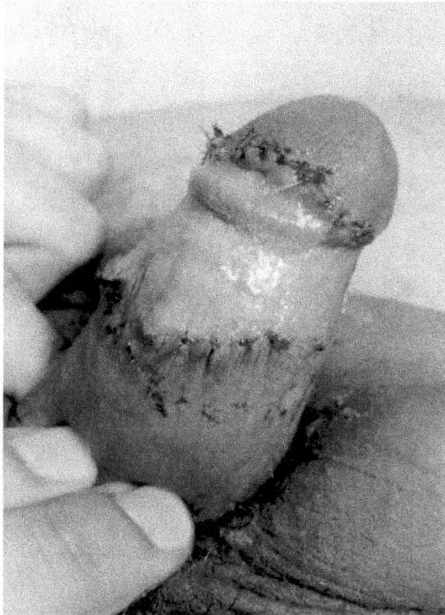

Figure 2.
Raw glans and an unappealing appearance of the glans resulting from the correction of large skin bridges.

6.3 Keloid formation

Any surgical procedure carries a risk of complications. Keloid scar formation is an abnormal proliferation of the scar extending beyond the surgical area. It is characterized by local fibroblast proliferation and overproduction of collagen. It sometimes takes a few months to develop. It is more common in younger individuals and is seen as more common in some ethnicities. Keloids cause cosmetic disfiguration, and the patient is usually bothered by the appearance of the scar. Genital keloid may cause functional impairment and worsen the quality of life. Keloids in the groin, especially those affecting the penis, are extremely rare despite frequent surgeries in the genital area. Only a few cases reported in the literature [41–45], hence the actual incidence is unknown.

Keloid formation is poorly understood. Numerous concepts have been suggested to understand the process by which keloid scars form. It has been suggested that keloid scars form as a result of collagen build-up, from the effect of hostile or hypoxic environment on tissue, or the hyperactivity of mast cells and the release of histamine. It has also been suggested that tension at scar edges create abnormal healing and might aid in the production of keloids [43].

Some topical therapies and therapeutic options have been described in the treatment of keloid scars. Treatments such as pressure on the keloid scar, silicone gel sheets, intralesional steroid injections, and massaging the scar with topical steroids have been suggested. A meta-analysis on the different treatment options for keloid scars has shown no statistical significance between the use of different treatment options separately or in combination [46]. Thus, no recognized guidelines have been established for the treatment of keloids. Surgical excision combined with intralesional steroid injections was and remained, the traditional treatment for keloids [47]. Creating a regulated treatment guideline has been challenging due to the lack of randomized controlled trials. The use of ablative laser technology, such as the CO2 laser, has lately produced hopeful outcomes.

6.4 Trauma

Although rare, traumatic complications of circumcisions have troubling consequences. Injury to the skin of the shaft [11, 48], injury to the glans or urethra [49–52], or total amputation of the whole length of the phallus are reported [53, 54]. These events, although very rare, are seen in rural regions where ritual mass circumcisions are performed by untrained individuals using primitive devices. They require referral to specialized centers with experience in reconstruction.

Circumcision, although it's considered to be a simple procedure, may cause serious problems such as penile skin necrosis or skin loss. Extensive skin removal is noticed at the end of the operation when the suture lines are under tension. Early postoperatively, the patients usually present with wound dehiscence after the first erection due to insufficient skin and stress on the suture line. Unfortunately, primary closure of such wound dehiscence is almost always unsuccessful. The skin is deficient, and skin stretch cannot accommodate the length of the erect penis; hence, another dehiscence is inevitable. If the penis is left to heal with secondary intention the scarring might entrap the penis, creating a buried penis. The scar of secondary intention might cause tethering or a mechanical pull on the erect penis. The bend of the penis might be painful; it might not permit a full erection to form and might hinder penetration and successful intercourse. The patient is left with frustration and grave disappointment, and the situation is left in the hands of the reconstructive urologists or plastic surgeons. Penile reconstructive surgery, in these cases, represents a significant challenge. The patient needs skin flaps or grafts from non-hair-bearing areas to cover the area of skin loss. The success of these procedures depends on the size of the area of skin loss, the use of flap vs. graft with its vascularity, and graft or flap take. Infection and excessive tension are the enemies in such cases and are to be prevented with all measures. A proper reconstruction procedure leaves the patient with excess skin that allows room for erection, has excellent visual appeal, is free of hair and contractions, and provides decent sensation. The use of scrotal-dartos-fascio-myo-cutaneous flap has been reported to cover up a defect of skin after circumcision procedure [48].

The penis is the organ which gives males their sexual confidence. Some of the devastating complications of circumcision are loss of part or the whole length of the penis. Trauma to the glans penis or even part of the penile shaft leaves behind a patient with low self-esteem and quality of life. Seleim and ElBarbany [22], after reviewing the literature, they did not find a grading system to define post-circumcision trauma to the penis. It was found that the term complete penile amputation, although obviously meant total penile loss, was used by authors to describe solitary glans amputation [55]. Therefore, they proposed a grading system to help better understand the extent of the injury, and to ease in finding the appropriate management options for each grade. Grade I was defined as skin complications, minor or major, ranging from simple skin infection or stitch sinus to major skin loss necessitating reconstruction. Grade II was for isolated urethral injury and the creation of an iatrogenic urethra-cutaneous fistula. Grade III was used to describe glans amputation and isolated glans injury. Grade IV was extended to include an insult to the corpora cavernosa. Grade V was defined as a total phallic loss either by amputation or gangrene [22]. All the patients in the study above had a history of circumcision being performed by inexperienced surgeons at primary care hospitals using electrocautery for hemostasis. This grading system helped in creating a standardized platform to help in understanding the extent of these injuries [20].

7. Conclusion

Circumcision is reported as one of the most common surgical procedures performed throughout the world. It is performed for religious reasons in Muslim and Jewish countries, for medical reasons such as phimosis or recurrent balanitis and are done electively for esthetic and cosmetic reasons. Unfortunately, it is still one of the most common rituals performed for religious reasons by inexperienced individuals. The incidence of complications of circumcision is quite low. It is believed to be a technically simple and safe surgical procedure. Having said that critical complications such as necrotizing fasciitis or total penile amputation may arise. Although circumcision is considered to be a technically simple and safe procedure with significantly low risk, it may occasionally lead to gravely devastating complications. It might place the patient in a state of mutilation, with low self-esteem. These complications present a reconstructive predicament, needing an expert in their repair. Even so, after the patch up work, the patient may still have psychological trauma and diminished sexual confidence.

Acknowledgements

Reem Aldamanhori is an associate professor in Imam Abdulrahman Bin Faisal University, Dammam, Saudi Arabia.

Conflict of interest

The author declares no conflict of interest.

Author details

Reem Aldamanhori
Imam Abdulrahman Bin Faisal University, Dammam, Saudi Arabia

*Address all correspondence to: rdamanhori@iau.edu.sa

IntechOpen

References

[1] Introcaso CE, Xu F, Kilmarx PH, Zaidi A, Markowitz LE. Prevalence of circumcision among men and boys aged 14 to 59 years in the United States, National Health and nutrition examination surveys 2005-2010. Sexually Transmitted Diseases. 2013;**40**(7):521-525

[2] Morris BJ, Kennedy SE, Wodak AD, Mindel A, Golovsky D, Schrieber L, et al. Early infant male circumcision: Systematic review, risk-benefit analysis, and progress in policy. World Journal of Clinical Pediatrics. 2017;**6**(1):89-102

[3] El Bcheraoui C, Zhang X, Cooper CS, Rose CE, Kilmarx PH, Chen RT. Rates of adverse events associated with male circumcision in U.S. medical settings, 2001 to 2010. JAMA Pediatrics. 2014;**168**(7):625-634

[4] Razzaq S, Mehmood MS, Tahir TH, Masood T, Ghaffar S. Safety of the plastibell circumcision in neonates, infants, and older children. International Journal of Health Sciences. 2018;**12**(5):10-13

[5] Horowitz M, Gershbein AB. Gomco circumcision: When is it safe? Journal of Pediatric Surgery. 2001;**36**(7):1047-1049

[6] Gerber JA, Borden AN, Broda J, Koelewyn S, Balasubramanian A, Tu D, et al. Evaluating clinical outcomes of an advanced practice provider-led newborn circumcision clinic. Urology. 2019;**127**:97-101

[7] Srinivasan M, Hamvas C, Coplen D. Rates of complications after newborn circumcision in a well-baby nursery, special care nursery, and neonatal intensive care unit. Clinical Pediatrics (Phila). 2015;**54**(12):1185-1191

[8] Kim JK, Koyle MA, Chua ME, Ming JM, Lee MJ, Kesavan A, et al. Assessment of risk factors for surgical complications in neonatal circumcision clinic. Canadian Urological Association Journal. 2019;**13**(4):E108-EE12

[9] Storm DW, Baxter C, Koff SA, Alpert S. The relationship between obesity and complications after neonatal circumcision. The Journal of Urology. 2011;**186**(Suppl 4):1638-1641

[10] Demaria J, Abdulla A, Pemberton J, Raees A, Braga LH. Are physicians performing neonatal circumcisions well-trained? Canadian Urological Association Journal. 2013;**7**(7-8):260-264

[11] İnce B, Dadacı M, Altuntaş Z, Bilgen F. Rarely seen complications of circumcision, and their management. Turkish Journal of Urology. 2016;**42**(1):12-15

[12] Peters JW, Schouw R, Anand KJ, van Dijk M, Duivenvoorden HJ, Tibboel D. Does neonatal surgery lead to increased pain sensitivity in later childhood? Pain. 2005;**114**(3):444-454

[13] Wang J, Zhao S, Luo L, Liu Y, Zhu Z, Li E, et al. Dorsal penile nerve block versus eutectic mixture of local anesthetics cream for pain relief in infants during circumcision: A meta-analysis. PLoS One. 2018;**13**(9):e0203439

[14] Kumar M, Chawla R, Goyal M. Topical anesthesia. Journal of Anaesthesiology Clinical Pharmacology. 2015;**31**(4):450-456

[15] Talini C, Antunes LA, Carvalho BCN, Schultz KL, Del Valle MHCP, Aranha Junior AA, et al. Circumcision: Postoperative complications that required reoperation. Einstein. 2018;**16**(3):eAO4241

[16] Bowa K, Li MS, Mugisa B, Waters E, Linyama DM, Chi BH, et al. A controlled trial of three methods

for neonatal circumcision in Lusaka, Zambia. Journal of Acquired Immune Deficiency Syndromes. 2013;**62**(1):e1-e6

[17] Raut A. Sutureless versus sutured circumcision: A comparative study. Urology Annals. 2019;**11**(1):87-90

[18] Voznesensky M, Mutter C, Hayn M, Kinkead T, Jumper B. Pediatric sutureless circumcision: An effective and cost efficient alternative. The Canadian Journal of Urology. 2015;**22**(5):7995-7999

[19] Akyüz O, Bodakçi MN, Tefekli AH. Thermal cautery-assisted circumcision and principles of its use to decrease complication rates. Journal of Pediatric Urology. 2019;**15**(2):186.e1-186.e8

[20] Al-Hazmi H, Traby M, Al-Yami F, Kattan AE, Al-Qattan MM. Penile reconstruction in a newborn following complicated circumcision: A case report. International Journal of Surgery Case Reports. 2018;**51**:74-77

[21] Fang DB, Shen YH, Zhu XW, Fang JJ, Mao QQ, Chao-jun W, et al. Penile necrosis resulting from post-circumcision microwave diathermy: A report of 9 cases. Zhonghua Nan Ke Xue. 2015;**21**(5):428-431

[22] Seleim HM, Elbarbary MM. Major penile injuries as a result of cautery during newborn circumcision. Journal of Pediatric Surgery. 2016;**51**(9):1532-1537

[23] Weiss HA, Larke N, Halperin D, Schenker I. Complications of circumcision in male neonates, infants and children: A systematic review. BMC Urology. 2010;**10**:2

[24] Heras A, Vallejo V, Pineda MI, Jacobs AJ, Cohen L. Immediate complications of elective newborn circumcision. Hospital Pediatrics. 2018;**8**(10):615-619

[25] Bastos Netto JM, de Araújo JG, de Almeida Noronha MF, Passos BR, de Bessa J, Figueiredo AA. Prospective randomized trial comparing dissection with Plastibell® circumcision. Journal of Pediatric Urology. 2010;**6**(6):572-577

[26] Baskin LS, Canning DA, Snyder HM, Duckett JW. Treating complications of circumcision. Pediatric Emergency Care. 1996;**12**(1):62-68

[27] Lebina L, Laher F, Mukudu H, Essien T, Otwombe K, Gray G, et al. Does routine prophylactic oral flucloxacillin reduce the incidence of post-circumcision infections? American Journal of Infection Control. 2013;**41**(10):897-900

[28] Galukande M, Sekavuga DB, Muganzi A, Coutinho A. Fournier's gangrene after adult male circumcision. International Journal of Emergency Medicine. 2014;7:37

[29] Scurlock JM, Pemberton PJ. Neonatal meningitis and circumcision. The Medical Journal of Australia. 1977;**1**(10):332-334

[30] Brook I. Infectious complications of circumcision and their prevention. European Urology Focus. 2016;**2**(4):453-459

[31] Frisch M, Simonsen J. Cultural background, non-therapeutic circumcision and the risk of meatal stenosis and other urethral stricture disease: Two nationwide register-based cohort studies in Denmark 1977-2013. The Surgeon. 2018;**16**(2):107-118

[32] Van Howe RS. Incidence of meatal stenosis following neonatal circumcision in a primary care setting. Clinical Pediatrics. 2006;**45**(1):49-54

[33] Morris BJ, Moreton S, Krieger JN. Meatal stenosis: Getting the diagnosis right. Research and Reports in Urology. 2018;**10**:237-239

[34] Karami H, Abedinzadeh M, Moslemi MK. Assessment of meatal stenosis in neonates undergoing circumcision using Plastibell device with two different techniques. Research and Reports in Urology. 2018;**10**:113-115

[35] Varda BK, Logvinenko T, Bauer S, Cilento B, Yu RN, Nelson CP. Minor procedure, major impact: Patient-reported outcomes following urethral meatotomy. Journal of Pediatric Urology. 2018;**14**(2):165.e1-165.e5

[36] Neheman A, Rappaport YH, Darawsha AE, Leibovitch I, Sternberg IA. Uroflowmetry before and after meatotomy in boys with symptomatic meatal stenosis following neonatal circumcision - a long-term prospective study. Urology. 2019;**125**:191-195

[37] Snodgrass W. Extensive skin bridging with glans epithelium replacement by penile shaft skin following newborn circumcision. Journal of Pediatric Urology. 2006;**2**(6):555-558

[38] Kampouroglou G, Nikas K. Penile skin bridges after circumcision. APSP Journal of Case Reports. 2015;**6**(3):33

[39] Kamal BA. Penile skin bridges: Causes and prevention. International Surgery. 2009;**94**(1):35-37

[40] Williams CP, Richardson BG, Bukowski TP. Importance of identifying the inconspicuous penis: Prevention of circumcision complications. Urology. 2000;**56**(1):140-142

[41] Xie LH, Li SK, Li Q. Combined treatment of penile keloid: A troublesome complication after circumcision. Asian Journal of Andrology. 2013;**15**(4):575-576

[42] Demirdover C, Sahin B, Vayvada H, Oztan HY. Keloid formation after circumcision and its treatment.

Journal of Pediatric Urology. 2013;**9**(1):e54-e56

[43] Alyami F, Ferandez N, Koyle MA, Salle JP. Keloid formation after pediatric male genital surgeries: An uncommon and difficult problem to manage. Journal of Pediatric Urology. 2019;**15**(1):48.e1-48.e8

[44] Ozakpinar HR, Sari E, Horoz U, Durgun M, Tellioglu AT, Acikgoz B. Keloid of the circumcision scar: A rare complication. International Wound Journal. 2015;**12**(5):611-612

[45] Park TH, Chang CH. Letter regarding "Keloid formation after circumcision and its treatment". Journal of Pediatric Urology. 2013;**9**(1):e56-e57

[46] Wong TS, Li JZ, Chen S, Chan JY, Gao W. The efficacy of triamcinolone acetonide in keloid treatment: A systematic review and meta-analysis. Frontiers in Medicine. 2016;**3**:71

[47] Heppt MV, Breuninger H, Reinholz M, Feller-Heppt G, Ruzicka T, Gauglitz GG. Current strategies in the treatment of scars and keloids. Facial Plastic Surgery. 2015;**31**(4):386-395

[48] Innocenti A, Tanini S, Mori F, Melita D, Innocenti M. Scrotal dartos-fascio-myo-cutaneous flaps for penis elongation after catastrophic iatrogenic skin shaft sub-amputation: A case of recovery using an extremely adaptable flap. International Journal of Surgery Case Reports. 2016;**28**:300-302

[49] Gluckman GR, Stoller ML, Jacobs MM, Kogan BA. Newborn penile glans amputation during circumcision and successful reattachment. The Journal of Urology. 1995;**153**(3 Pt 1): 778-779

[50] Giovanny A, Wahyudi I, Rodjani A. Neo-glans reconstruction after glans amputation during circumcision using autologous buccal

mucosal graft. Urology Case Reports.
2018;**18**:11-13

[51] Khaireddine B, Adnen H, Khaled BM,
Adel S. Surgical reimplantation of
penile glans amputation in children
during circumcision. Urology Annals.
2014;**6**(1):85-87

[52] Baskin LS, Canning DA, Snyder HM,
Duckett JW. Surgical repair of urethral
circumcision injuries. The Journal of
Urology. 1997;**158**(6):2269-2271

[53] van der Merwe A, Graewe F,
Zühlke A, Barsdorf NW, Zarrabi AD,
Viljoen JT, et al. Penile allotransplan-
tation for penis amputation following
ritual circumcision: A case report
with 24 months of follow-up. Lancet.
2017;**390**(10099):1038-1047

[54] Kim JH, Park JY, Song YS. Traumatic
penile injury: From circumcision injury
to penile amputation. BioMed Research
International. 2014;**2014**:375285

[55] Hashem FK, Ahmed S, al-Malaq AA,
AbuDaia JM. Successful replantation of
penile amputation (post-circumcision)
complicated by prolonged ischaemia.
British Journal of Plastic Surgery.
1999;**52**(4):308-310

Chapter 5

Male Circumcision and Infection

Ruth Mielke

Abstract

Worldwide, male circumcision is done for religious or cultural reasons, and to a lesser degree for medical indications. Newborn male circumcision is associated with fewer genitourinary infections in younger males. In the current decade, a substantial body of research suggests that male circumcision is effective as a prophylactic measure against HIV and other sexually transmitted infections. The compelling HIV reductions in 3 African randomized control trials in circumcised men have prompted use of male circumcision as a key part of HIV prevention in developing nations. More recently, the use of male circumcision as a public health measure in developed nations is a topic of international discussion.

Keywords: male circumcision, sexually transmitted infections, sexually transmitted diseases, HIV, urinary tract infection, HPV

1. Introduction

Historically, male circumcision has been done for religious/cultural reasons and to a lesser degree, for medical indications. Contemporary discussion of male circumcision relates to its utility as a public health measure – specifically in the prevention of genitourinary and sexually transmitted infections. Male circumcision was suggested to prevent sexually transmitted infection as early as the 1850s [1] and broadly as a "sanitary measure" in 1914 [2]. However, when three large randomized controlled trials in sub-Sahara Africa reported that male circumcision reduced the risk of acquiring HIV infection in males by as much as 60%, [3–5] attention to its health benefits became a world-wide discussion. In 2007, the World Health Organization (WHO), and the Joint United Nations Programme on HIV/AIDS (UNAIDS), announced that male circumcision was integral to comprehensive HIV prevention [6, 7].

Most professional organizations in developed nations do not recommended routine use of newborn male circumcision but recognize its use in disease prevention. The American Urological Association, Canadian Paediatric Society, Canadian Urological Association and Royal Australasian College of Physicians recognize a benefit for some boys in high-risk populations [8–11]. However, the Centers for Disease Control supports infant and later age MC and the American Academy of Pediatrics endorses newborn MC; e.g. "current evidence indicates that the health benefits of newborn male circumcision outweigh the risks, and the benefits of newborn male circumcision justify access to this procedure for those families who choose it" [12, 13].

This chapter will discuss the impact of male circumcision in the context of the health promotion and health prevention specific to genitourinary and sexually transmitted infections.

2. Physiology of the foreskin

Male circumcision involves cutting and removing all or part of the foreskin, or prepuce, from the glans penis. To understand the rationale for the use of male circumcision (MC) in prevention of infections, it is important to understand the function and physiology of the foreskin. At birth, the glans penis and inner foreskin share a common, fused mucosal epithelium called the balano-preputial lamina (BPL). Much like the membrane that fuses the fingernail to the finger, it acts as "living glue". The extent of this fusion is such that the foreskin can only be retracted in 4% of newborn boys resulting in physiologic phimosis; natural inability to separate the foreskin. As the penis grows in the first 3–4 years of the boy's life, the foreskin gradually separates from the glans when smegma, epithelial debris produced by sebaceous glands, accumulates under the foreskin [14]. By age 10 most boys have a retractable foreskin, and by age 17, natural separation of the foreskin from the glans penis is complete [15] (**Figure 1**).

2.1 Uncircumcised

There are divergent viewpoints on the purpose and function of the foreskin. MC opponents view the keratinized squamous epithelium that covers the penile shaft and the foreskin in the uncircumcised penis as having protective functions. Beyond being epithelial debris, smegma is a natural emollient that protects and lubricates the glans. One author's suggestion that the inner foreskin contains apocrine glands that secrete substances e.g. lysozymes and cytokines with antibacterial properties [16] has not been verified in biochemical research. It is contended that neonatal male circumcision not only removes tissue containing fine-touch receptors but interferes with the natural separation process. This may lead to subsequent sensory imbalance and risk of injury and tears that make the circumcised penis less hygienic and more prone to infection [17].

2.2 Circumcised

The alternate view is that the biochemical and structural properties of the intact foreskin result in increased acquisition of HIV and other STIs. During intercourse, the foreskin slides backward and exposes the inner mucosal surface with its high density of target cells for HIV, Langerhans cells, CD4+ cells, and macrophages - providing an entry point for pathogens. Lymphoid areas of mucosal surfaces are primary sites for HIV infection. Foreskin tissue has been identified as both having abundant HIV target cells and susceptibility to trauma because of its thinly keratinized surface [18]. Structurally, the folding of the foreskin on the non-erect

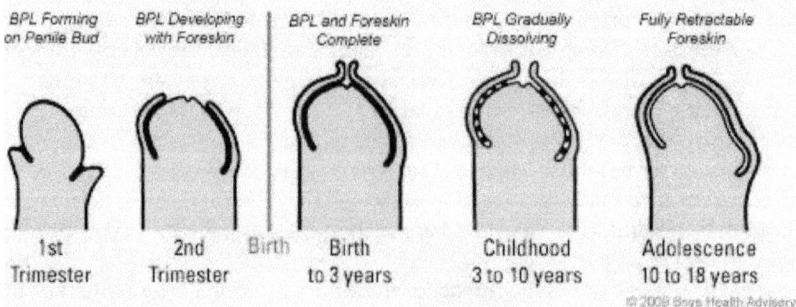

Figure 1.
Physiologic changes in the male foreskin and balano-preputial lamina (BPL) over time.

uncircumcised penis creates a sub-preputial space which is eliminated on the erect penis. By removing the foreskin surgically, this space is eliminated thereby removing the reservoir for HIV, human papilloma virus (HPV), and other pathogens [19–21]. In theory, removal of the foreskin HIV reduces target cells, eliminates the sticky medium for viruses, exposes the more keratinized penile shaft and eliminates the sub-preputial space which collectively diminishes pathogen exposure.

3. Urinary tract infection

Urinary tract infection (UTI) is one of the more common bacterial infections in children with 1–3% of children experiencing one UTI in early childhood [22, 23]. The strongest risk factors are renal tract abnormalities, which are relatively rare [24]. Common risk factors are female gender, young age, and uncircumcised state in boys [22, 25, 26]. A population study in Australia (N = 2856), conducted over 12.8 years in which most males (80.7%) were uncircumcised, reported the prevalence of UTI as twice (5.3%) in girls than in boys (2.1%) [25]. An epidemiologic study of 596 cases of childhood UTI in Sweden, where circumcision is uncommon, reported the prevalence of UTI by 11 years of age to be 3.0% for girls and 1.1% for boys. [23] Other sex differences observed by were that the prevalence of UTI was highest during the first month of life and then decreased more rapidly in boys than in girls [23, 27]. As the uncircumcised foreskin may support the growth of pathogenic bacteria at the meatus [28], this decline in UTI prevalence in boys likely occurred because of the physiologic retraction of the prepuce over time [16].

3.1 Current research

The associations of MC and UTI in older studies were limited due to having samples with disproportionately larger groups of circumcised boys and generally, because of being single studies of observational, non-experimental design. More robust evidence of the disease prevention potential of MC with respect to UTI has come about from more recent multi-study reviews [26, 29]. One of these, a meta-analysis of 22 studies (21 observational and one randomized controlled trial of 70 participants) examined lack of circumcision as a risk factor for UTI and reported a lifetime relative risk of UTI as 3.7 times higher than that in uncircumcised males. Stratified for age, the risk of UTI was 9.91 greater for those aged 0–1 year; 6.56 greater for those aged 1–16 years; and 3.41 for those older than 16 years, in uncircumcised males [26]. These results are consistent with the known decline of UTIs in males as they mature, but also suggest that the effect of MC in UTI prevention is most evident in infants and younger boys.

3.2 High-risk populations

Recurrent UTIs are the principal cause of permanent kidney tissue scarring in children, so interventions that reduce frequency of UTIs are needed to prevent short and long-term morbidity. Vesicoureteral reflux (VUR), an abnormal retrograde or "back" flow of urine from the bladder to the upper urinary tract, is the most common abnormality of the urinary tract in children and is found in 30–40% of children with UTI [30]. In children with VUR, risk of UTI recurrence increases to 10 and 30% [31]. One review of 12 studies (one RCT, 4 cohort studies, and 7 case-control studies) used a meta-analysis to assess the effect of MC on UTI, and then estimated the degree of benefit in normal boys compared to those with (a) recurrent UTI and (b) VUR, who have increased risk of UTI. Male circumcision was associated with a significantly reduced risk (87%) of UTI [31]. However, given the low risk of UTI in normal boys (1%) they estimated that the number of MC needed to prevent one UTI was 111. However, in higher risk boys, the number of MC needed to treat those with recurrent UTIs was reduced to 11 and for those with VUR to 4 [31]. This suggests that use of MC particularly in higher risk groups of boys is an intervention to reduce UTI, subsequent renal scarring and loss of renal reserve.

Prenatal hydronephrosis (fetal urinary tract dilatation), is one of the most common congenital urological anomalies, and is reported in 1–2% of all pregnancies [32]. Prenatal identification of high-grade hydronephrosis has been associated with VUR and 3-fold increase in UTIs, so such findings may warrant consideration of early infant male circumcision [33]. Genetics has increasing importance in identifying those at risk for recurrent UTI. Genes have been identified that cause inefficient bacterial clearance and greater susceptibility to UTIs [34]. Syndromes in which there are genital tract anomalies, most prominently, vesicoureteral reflux, may increase the risk for recurrent UTI [24, 32, 33]. Early infant male circumcision (EIMC) may be warranted in boys who are at risk for recurrent UTIs based on prenatal findings.

4. Sexually transmitted infections

Worldwide, more than 1 million sexually transmitted infections (STIs) are acquired daily [35, 36]. Organisms causing STIs are bacterial, protozoal, and viral. Those with bacterial (chlamydia, gonorrhea, syphilis) or protozoal (trichomonas) causes are treatable while those caused by viruses (herpes simplex, human papilloma, HIV) are not [36, 37]. Each year, 376 million new infections are caused by chlamydia, gonorrhea, syphilis and trichomonas and more than 500 million persons experience genital infections from herpes simplex virus (HSV) [36, 38] (**Figure 2**). Most STIs have no symptoms or only mild symptoms that may not be recognized as an STI. Further, STIs such as HSV type 2 and syphilis increase the risk of HIV acquisition. Longer term, STIs can have serious reproductive health consequences beyond the immediate impact of the infection such as infertility, mother-to-child transmission and genitourinary cancers. Moreover, people with sexually transmitted infections often experience stigma, stereotyping, vulnerability, shame and gender-based violence [35].

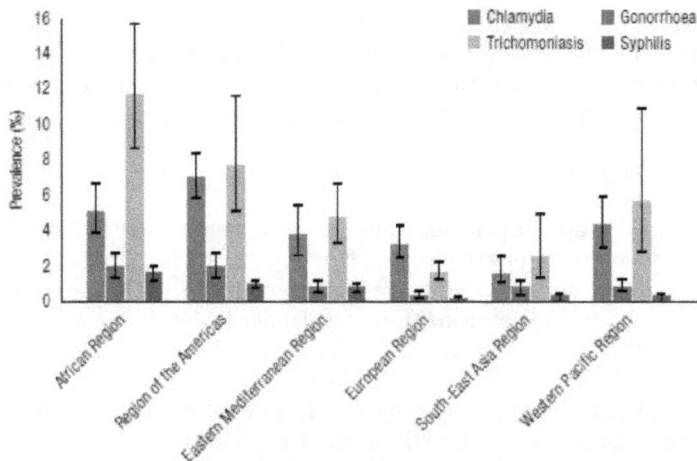

Figure 2.
Estimated prevalence of chlamydia, gonorrhea, trichomoniasis and active syphilis in women aged 15–49 years by WHO region, 2009–2016 Source: WHO Report on global sexually transmitted infection surveillance, 2018.

4.1 HIV

The health burden of HIV infections is greatest in developing countries where HIV is more prevalent, and treatment is least available. **Figure 3** shows geographic extremes ranging from 0.1% to nearly 5% in Africa. Of the 39.3 million persons living with HIV worldwide, nearly 70% live in Sub-Saharan Africa [39]. Of those, adolescent girls and women account for a disproportionate percentage (59%) of new HIV infections among adults aged 15 and older. This contrasts with other parts of the world, where men account for 63% of the new adult HIV infections. Globally, there were almost 90,000 more new HIV infections among men than women in 2017 [40]. Therefore, reaching more men with HIV treatment but more proactively, with preventive measures such as circumcision, is critical to breaking cycles of HIV transmission and reducing HIV incidence among young women. If fewer men acquire HIV because of male circumcision, this will benefit women by reducing exposure to HIV-infected men.

4.1.1 Heterosexual transmission

The potential of male circumcision to protect from heterosexual HIV infection was first suggested in 1986 [41]. Subsequently, a rich body of research done in developing countries has emerged focusing on the relationship between male circumcision and heterosexual HIV acquisition in men. In a review of (1) biological evidence, (2) observational study data supported by high-quality meta-analyses, and the (3) results of three well-recognized randomized clinical trials [3–5] (**Table 1**) and high-quality meta-analyses [42, 43] from 1999 to 2011, all of the highest quality studies; Grades 1 and 2 (meta-analyses and randomized control trials) favored MC in terms of reducing HIV risk as did the vast majority of the Grades 3 and 4 (case-control/observational studies and expert opinion) studies [44].

A more recent meta-analysis evaluated the effect of male circumcision on HIV acquisition for HIV (−/+) males and HIV (−) females during heterosexual behavior. The analysis of fifteen studies (4 RCTs and 11 prospective cohort) reported strong evidence that male circumcision was associated with reduced HIV acquisition for HIV (−)

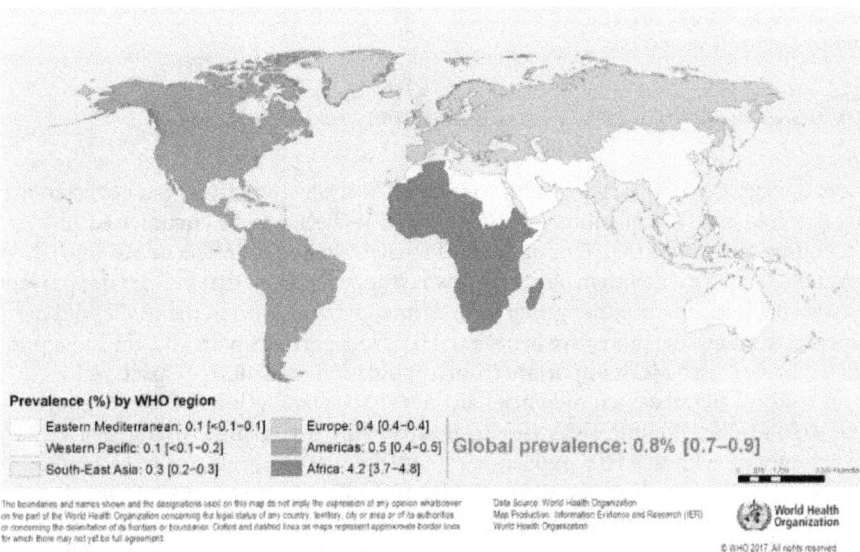

Prevalence (%) by WHO region

Eastern Mediterranean: 0.1 [<0.1–0.1] Europe: 0.4 [0.4–0.4]
Western Pacific: 0.1 [<0.1–0.2] Americas: 0.5 [0.4–0.5] Global prevalence: 0.8% [0.7–0.9]
South-East Asia: 0.3 [0.2–0.3] Africa: 4.2 [3.7–4.8]

The boundaries and names shown and the designations used on this map do not imply the expression of any opinion whatsoever on the part of the World Health Organization concerning the legal status of any country, territory, city or area or of its authorities, or concerning the delimitation of its frontiers or boundaries. Dotted and dashed lines on maps represent approximate border lines for which there may not yet be full agreement.

Data Source: World Health Organization
Map Production: Information Evidence and Research (IER)
World Health Organization

World Health Organization

© WHO 2017. All rights reserved.

Figure 3.
Prevalence of HIV among adults aged 15 to 49, 2016 by WHO region.

Male circumcision and HIV and STI acquisition in men and transmission to female partners			
	Ratio (95% confidence interval) by study location[a]		
	Uganda	South Africa	Kenya
	N = 4996	N = 3274	N = 2784
Male protection benefit			
HIV	0.43 (0.24–0.75)[b]	0.40 (0.24–0.68)[b]	0.47 (0.28–0.78)[b]
High-risk HPV	0.65 (0.46–0.90)[c]	0.68 (0.52–0.89)[c]	
HSV-2	0.72 (0.56–0.92)[d]	0.66 (0.32–1.12)[b]	
Syphilis	1.10 (0.75–1.65)[d]		
Neisseria gonorrhoeae		0.87 (0.60–1.26)[c]	0.95 (0.68–1.34)[b]
Chlamydia trachomatis		0.56 (0.32–1.00)[e]	0.87 (0.65–1.16)[b]
Trichomonas vaginalis		0.53 (0.28–1.02)[e]	0.77 (0.44–1.36)[b]
GUD	0.53 (0.43–0.64)[c]		
Female protection benefit			
HIV	1.49 (0.62–3.57)[d]		
Bacterial vaginosis (any)	0.60 (0.38–0.94)[c]		
Bacterial vaginosis (severe)	0.39 (0.24–0.64)[c]		
Trichomonas vaginalis	0.52 (0.05–0.98)[c]		
GUD	0.78 (0.63–0.97)[c]		
High-risk HPV	0.72 (0.60–0.85)[c]		

Adapted with permission of John Wiley and Sons.
Abbreviations: GUD, genital ulcer disease; HIV, human immunodeficiency virus; HPV, human papillomavirus;
HSV-2, herpes simplex virus type 2; STI, sexually transmitted infection.
[a]*Data shown are from 3 randomized controlled trials by Gray et al. [5], Auvert et al. [3], and Bailey et al. [4], that
presented the effect of male circumcision on HIV/STI acquisition in men, 2 RCTs and a secondary analysis related to
the Ugandan study on effect of MC in HIV (−/+) men on female partners by Wawer et al. [46], MC effect on HPV
acquisition in female partners by Wawer et al. [60], and a MC effect on female partner STI acquisition by Gray
et al. [85]. All ratios are adjusted (except for South African HSV-2 and Kenyan bacterial STIs) and represent an
intention-to-treat analysis.*
[b]*The ratio expressed is an incidence rate ratio.*
[c]*The ratio expressed is a prevalence risk ratio.*
[d]*The ratio expressed is a hazard ratio.*
[e]*The ratio expressed is an odds ratio.*

Table 1.
Male circumcision and HIV and STI acquisition in men and transmission to female partners.

males during sexual intercourse with females (70% protective effect) but no difference
was detected in HIV acquisition for HIV (−) females between the circumcised and
uncircumcised groups [45]. One of the RCTs that evaluated the effect of MC in HIV
(+) and (−) men on their female partners was stopped early in that MC did not prevent
female HIV infection in either group [46]. Although the women in the studies did not
experience individual protective benefit of HIV from partners with MC, the reduction
of HIV in men with MC is important from a population reduction perspective.

A study of heterosexual men in a Baltimore, Maryland (United States) reported
that 1096 (2.7%) of clinic visits yielded positive HIV test results. Among 394 visits
by patients with known HIV exposure, circumcision was significantly associated
with lower HIV prevalence (10.2 vs. 22.0%) [87]. This suggests that MC may have a
role in HIV prevention in resource rich countries as well.

The optimal time for MC is when the man is HIV (−) but there may be benefit in
HIV (+) men as well. WHO/UNAIDS have recommended that MC not be denied to

HIV-infected men who request the procedure (unless there are medical contraindications) to reduce stigma but also as MC can reduce acquisition of HPV in men and syphilis and herpes in their female partners [47–49]. Further, including all males in voluntary medical male circumcision programs, irrespective of HIV status, results in greater population uptake as higher risk HIV (−) males who may otherwise avoid programs due to fear of being tested for HIV will be more likely to participate [50]. In an RCT of HIV-positive men in Uganda, MC did not reduce HIV transmission to women over a period of 2 years [48]. However, the higher rate of HIV transmission in couples who initiated intercourse soon after MC compared to those who waited until healing occurred, underscores the importance of delaying intercourse until the MC wound is healed.

Therefore, MC protects men from HIV infection in areas where prevalence of HIV (e.g. sub-Saharan Africa) is high, is largely due to heterosexual transmission, and where access to antivirals is low. Male circumcision does not appear to decrease HIV acquisition in their female partners on an individual level but decreasing new HIV infections overall will ultimately reduce the HIV burden in the population overall.

4.1.2 Homosexual transmission

The case for MC as a preventive measure is less compelling in areas where HIV acquisition is largely due to men who have sex with men. In developed countries, where HIV prevalence overall is low, most HIV are cases are related to homosexual transmission e.g. in the United States, 66%, [51, 52]. Further, developed countries have access to antivirals for prevention as well as for treatment of HIV infection which keep prevalence of new infections and AIDs mortality low. One review of 20 observational studies (N = 71,693), reported that the pooled effect estimate for HIV acquisition in homosexual men was not statistically significant. However, when subgroups were analyzed, the results of 7 studies of men reporting an insertive role were statistically significant for a 27% reduction in HIV acquisition in contrast to the 3 studies of men reporting a receptive role [53]. However, a more recent meta-analysis by Sharma et al. that examined the impact of sexual roles among homosexual men reported that MC did not definitively have a protective effect among predominantly insertive homosexual men or receptive men but acknowledged that there were a small number of studies reporting the effect of sexual role on HIV acquisition [54].

More broadly, the Sharma et al. meta-analysis of 49 studies was conducted to assess MC as a method to prevent HIV acquisition in homosexual and/or heterosexual men. The overall pooled risk ratio (RR) for both homosexual and heterosexual men was 0.58 (95% CI 0.48–0.70), suggesting that MC was associated with a reduction in HIV risk. Heterosexual men had a greater risk reduction (72%) compared with 20% for homosexual men. However, there was significant heterogeneity among the studies and less than 6% of total subject count was from randomized controlled trials [54]. Although the study suggests that MC was effective in reducing HIV risk for both heterosexual and homosexual men, the effect was dramatically lower in homosexual men.

Male circumcision represents one of very few proven HIV prevention strategies particularly in high prevalence areas, such as sub-Saharan Africa where transmission is largely related to heterosexual contact. It is less clear whether voluntary male medical circumcision programs, such as those employed in Africa would be as beneficial in developed nations. In the United States, HIV prevalence is comparatively low and most new HIV infections are attributed to men having sex with men. Theoretically, certain groups in the United States, e.g. African-American and Hispanic men with higher risk of HIV infections could benefit but this impact would be much less profound [12]. In addition, the reality that individuals may identify as either homosexual or heterosexual but are bisexually active further confounds the potential effect of MC on homosexual transmission of HIV.

4.2 Human papilloma virus

Human papillomavirus (HPV) has been established as the leading cause of invasive cervical cancer in women and is associated with anogenital warts and cancers in men and women [55]. Of the 100+ strains of HPV; about 40 affect the anogenital areas. HPV strains are classified as either low-risk (causes benign lesions) or high-risk (causes malignancies). Oncogenic high-risk strains (e.g. HPV types 16 and 18) cause most of the HPV-related cancers and pre-cancers, while the low-risk strains cause genital warts or mild Pap test abnormalities. Most sexually active persons will contract HPV infection at some time in their lives but in most cases, the infection will be asymptomatic and clear spontaneously. Risk factors associated with HPV infection include, increased exposure to the virus via multiple partners, decreased condom usage, history of other STIs, tobacco usage, and for women, having sex with an uncircumcised partner [56].

4.2.1 HPV in women

More than 290 million women have human papillomavirus (HPV) infection [57]. Worldwide, cervical cancer is the fourth most frequent cancer in women and fourth leading cause of death in women. In developing countries, cervical cancer ranks second (breast cancer is first) in incidence and mortality. Approximately 90% of deaths from cervical cancer occur in low- and middle-income countries where women do not have access to pap testing and HPV vaccine [58, 59]. Absent of such health resources, MC in their partners provides a means of HPV prevention and exposure reduction for women.

A challenge to ascertaining associations between a woman's HPV risk and her partner's circumcision status is the reality that she may have numerous partners in her lifetime. A study of HPV and cervical cancer in women with only one male partner demonstrated HPV infection of 5.5% in circumcised versus 19.6% of uncircumcised men [19]. Therefore, the procedure of MC itself removes a reservoir for viruses, such as HPV, thus reducing exposure over the long-term.

As the precursor of cervical cancer, reducing high-risk HPV transmission is a critical part of disease prevention. Decreased prevalence of high-risk HPV was found in an RCT of Ugandan women whose long-term partners were circumcised immediately compared with women with partners who were circumcised 24 months after enrollment [60] (**Table 1**). The significant reduction (28%) in high-risk HPV that was observed in women whose partners were circumcised earlier suggests that MC has a role in reducing HPV exposure to women in areas where HPV vaccine is not readily available.

A systematic review by Grund et al. analyzed data from 60 studies on the influence MC on women's health outcomes [47]. In the cervical cancer and cervical dysplasia groups, there were no RCTs, but the quality of the studies was graded using the Newcastle-Ottawa scale for non-randomized studies. All but one of the studies reported a highly protective effect of MC related to cervical cancer (in the exception study only 11% of the men were circumcised) [61]. In the same review, four of the five cases reviewed also showed that MC was highly protective of cervical dysplasia and moderately protective of HPV infection. In developed countries, access to HPV vaccination along with early identification and treatment of cervical dysplasia is a well-established part of preventive health care for women. In resource poor countries without such preventive care programs, the protective effect of MC on cervical dysplasia and cancer offers a critical means of preventing morbidity and mortality in women.

4.2.2 HPV in men

HPV is the most common STI in the world. More attention has been on HPV infection in women because of its association with cervical cancer. In men, manifestations of HPV infection range from genital warts and mild dysplasia (low-risk strains) to rarely, anogenital cancers (high-risk strains). Two of the African trials [3, 5] (**Table 1**) reported that MC was associated with an estimated 33% reduced occurrence of high-risk HPV virus in men. Two reviews and meta-analyses analyzed the effect of male circumcision on genital HPV infection in men. Albero et al. (21 studies; N = 14,382) reported that MC was associated with a 43% reduction in both low- and high-risk strains of HPV and in two studies (RCTs), 33% reduction in high-risk HPV. However, no associations were found in the acquisition of new HPV infections, genital HPV clearance, or genital warts [62]. Larke et al. (27 studies; N = 10,779) also reported that MC was associated with modest (25%) HPV reduction but no evidence of an association with genital warts [63]. However, Larke et al. reported 33% increased HPV clearance after MC which is important when considering that diminishing viral load in men reduces exposure to their female partners.

Penile cancer is rare—globally with 0.84 cases per 100,000 person-years [64]. High-risk HPV infection has a considerable role in penile cancer, but with less consistency than in cervical cancer. In contrast to cervical cancer, in which HPV is responsible for nearly all cases, HPV infection is associated with penile cancer from 55 to 82% of the time [65]. In a study of HIV-positive men in Uganda, MC reduced the prevalence and incidence of multiple HR-HPV infections. Multiple HR-HPV infections were found in 22.4% of subjects in the intervention (MC) group and in 42.5% of those in the control (no MC) group demonstrating 47% efficacy [48]. Therefore, male circumcision may provide a direct benefit for HIV-positive men by preventing penile HR-HPV infection and thus potentially averting penile cancer. In addition, it is possible that circumcision of HIV-infected men may protect female partners from infection and potentially from cervical neoplasia.

5. Other sexually transmitted infections

Male circumcision has a role in the acquisition of other sexually transmitted infections. Although MC has not been directly associated with decreases in HIV transmission to female partners [5] (**Table 1**) it is still important to understand whether MC affects ulcerative sexually transmitted infections such as HSV type 2 [66–68] and syphilis [67, 69] both of which are associated with an increased risk of HIV.

5.1 Herpes simplex virus

Infection with the herpes simplex virus (HSV) is due to herpes simplex virus type 1 (HSV-1) or herpes simplex virus type 2 (HSV-2). HSV-1 is mainly transmitted by oral contact to cause infection in or around the mouth (oral herpes). HSV-2 is almost exclusively sexually transmitted, causing infection in the genital or anal area (genital herpes) [70]. HSV infection is highly stigmatized and negatively impacts relationships. However, more critical is its potential for perinatal transmission, resulting newborn morbidity and mortality [71–73] and its well-documented relationship with HIV.

Perinatal transmission mostly occurs during delivery from mothers with herpes simplex virus HSV-1 or HSV-2 genital infection. If contracted, 60% of newborns will die without treatment [73]. In a first estimate of global neonatal herpes infection, Looker et al. reported 14,000 neonatal herpes cases annually and that most neonatal herpes cases occurred in Africa, due to high maternal HSV-2 infection and high birth rates. HSV-1 contributed more cases than HSV-2 in the Americas, Europe, and Western Pacific [72]. Therefore, understanding the relationship between MC and HSV transmission is important as circumcision may afford important benefit in terms of reductions in HSV infections, particularly in female partners in their childbearing years.

HSV-2 is a leading cause of genital ulcer disease worldwide, but prevalence by global region differs [71]. Looker et al. reported that Africa had the highest prevalence (32%), followed by the Americas (14%), with Africa contributing most to the global totals due to combined large population and high prevalence. Despite their lower prevalence, South-East Asia (8%) and Western Pacific (8%) also contributed large numbers infected to the global totals due to their large population numbers [38].

Women are more likely to acquire HSV-2 than men and certain ethnicities are at greater risk. For instance in the United States, the prevalence of HSV-2 in adults is 12.1%; but affects women (15.9%) more so than men (8.2%) and is highest among non-Hispanic black persons (34.6%) [74]. In Africa, HSV-2 prevalence in men ranged from 5.9 to 39.8% while in women, from 29.2% (rural women) to 79.9% (sex workers) [75].

Two of the African RCTs reported that MC was associated with HSV-2 reductions of 28 and 34% in men [3, 5] (**Table 1**). Subsequently, a large meta-analysis (N = 49) supported this original finding with respect to HSV reductions in men in that MC diminished risk of HSV-2 by 15% and genital ulcers (often due to HSV-2) by 20% [54]. There are fewer reports of the relationship between MC and HSV infections in the female partners. However, in the Grund et al. systematic review of MC and women's health outcomes, the direction of the evidence in the six studies (including one RCT) was highly protective of HSV-2 [47]. Five of the studies were in developing countries and one was in the U.S. suggesting greater global generalizability.

The HIV epidemic in sub-Saharan Africa is known to be fueled by HSV-2 consequently directing attention on the prevalence and transmission of HSV-2 in in recent years [68, 75]. Abu-Rabbad et al. estimated that in areas of high HSV-2 prevalence, such as Kisumu, Kenya, more than a quarter of incident HIV infections may have been attributed directly to HSV-2 [68]. Therefore, the role of MC in reducing HSV-2 transmission has the potential for short-term benefit along with long-term influence in perinatal health promotion and disease prevention.

5.2 Syphilis

Syphilis can cause neurological, cardiovascular and dermatological disease in adults, and stillbirth, neonatal death, premature delivery or severe disability in infants [36]. Women of childbearing age are a particularly vulnerable population. During pregnancy, the immunosuppression of pregnancy increases risk of syphilis acquisition and if untreated or undertreated, there is great risk for adverse infant consequences. In 2016, 988,000 pregnant women worldwide were infected with syphilis, resulting in over 350,000 such adverse outcomes including 200,000 stillbirths and newborn deaths [76].

The interaction between syphilis and HIV is complex and continues to be studied [69]. The World Health Organization has identified dual elimination of HIV and syphilis as a global health priority [77]. In the early stages of syphilis, painless genital sores (chancres or ulcers) facilitate transmission of HIV infection sexually. Conversely, the immunocompromised state of HIV infection makes syphilis acquisition more likely. In developed countries, homosexual (men having sex with men) are the largest affected group [78, 79]. However, recent increases in congenital syphilis in developed [78] and developing countries warrant attention to the learning the potential value of MC in prevention of syphilis acquisition in women as well.

Several reviews have studied the influence of MC and syphilis. Weiss et al. studied risk of three ulcerative STIs (syphilis, chancroid, and genital herpes) and reported that of the syphilis studies (N = 14), there was substantial reduction of syphilis (33%) in men; however, this was limited by significant heterogeneity between the studies. The reduced risk of HSV-2 infection was of borderline statistical significance and MC was associated with lower risk of chancroid in six of seven studies [80]. More recently, a large review (N = 60) of studies assessed the association between MC and women's health outcomes included six studies on syphilis acquisition [47]. All the studies were in developing countries; there were no RCTs. The results were that MC was highly protective; all studies reported a reduction in syphilis with one reporting no cases of syphilis in the treatment (MC) group [81].

Partners PrEP Study Team followed 4716 HIV sero-discordant couples, of whom roughly 50% of the men were circumcised. During the follow-up period (~ 2·75 years), MC was associated with significantly fewer cases of syphilis by 42% in men compared with uncircumcised men and was most protective for HIV (+) men as demonstrated by 62% reduction. Further, MC male circumcision reduced overall female partner syphilis incidence by 59%; by 75% in the HIV (−) women and a 48% HIV (+) women. Thus, MC was strongly associated with reductions in syphilis acquisition in both men and their female partners. This suggests that MC decreases syphilis acquisition even in HIV discordant couples and should be an option for HIV (+) men in countries employing voluntary medical male circumcision to reduce syphilis [77, 82].

5.3 Genital ulcerative disease

Genital ulcerative disease (GUD) is associated with an increased risk of HIV acquisition and transmission. The ulcer results from various sexually transmitted infections but the ulcer's disruption of the skin tissue promotes co-infection by other viruses and bacteria. In the United States most genital ulcers are due to HSV or syphilis. Less prevalent infectious causes include chancroid (*Haemophilus ducreyi*), granuloma inguinale (*Klebsiella granulomatis*), and lymphogranuloma venereum [83].

Lymphogranuloma venereum (LGV) is a sexually transmitted infection caused by certain chlamydia trachomatis strains. LGV is common in certain areas of Africa, Southeast Asia, India, the Caribbean, and South America. It is rare in developed countries, but in the last 10 years has been increasingly recognized in North America, Europe, and the United Kingdom as causing rectal infections among men who have sex with men [84]. In the Ugandan RCT, MC reduced the risk of genital ulcer disease (GUD) in men by 50% [5] (**Table 1**).

5.4 Gonorrhea, chlamydia, trichomonas, and bacterial vaginosis infections

These bacterial STIs cause cervicitis, urethritis, vaginitis and genital ulceration, and some may also infect the rectum and pharynx. Chlamydia and gonorrhea are associated with serious short- and long-term conditions such as pelvic inflammatory disease, ectopic pregnancy, infertility, chronic pelvic pain and arthritis. They also can be transmitted to the newborn infant during pregnancy or delivery [36].

The three African RCTs also reported associations between MC and gonorrhea, chlamydia, trichomonas, and bacterial vaginosis (**Table 1**). The South African trial reported reductions with borderline statistical significance in male acquisition of chlamydia (44%) and trichomonas (47%) in men with MC [3]. The Kenyan study results suggested reductions in chlamydia and trichomonas, but neither was statistically significant [4]. Neither study reported an association between MC and gonorrhea in men. Gray reported statistically significant reductions in bacterial vaginosis (any severity) (40%), severe bacterial vaginosis (61%) and trichomonas (48%) in females whose partners had MC [85].

Grund et. al's review of the impact of MC on women's health outcomes reported high quality evidence that MC was protective of chlamydia, that effect was moderately generalizable, and inclusive of studies from Africa, Americas, Asia, Europe and the U.S. In contrast, low consistency evidence was found for MC and female acquisition of trichomonas, bacterial vaginosis, and gonorrhea [47].

6. Summary and conclusions

Three African trials of male circumcision in HIV-negative men showed that circumcision reduced male acquisition of HIV by 50–60%. As a result, male

Male Circumcision and Infection - Information to Share
1. Consider factors associated with decision making
Health benefits and risks of elective neonatal, adolescent, or adult medically performed male circumcision should be considered in consultation with medical providers while considering factors associated with decision-making around male circumcision, including religion, societal norms and social customs, hygiene, aesthetic preference, and ethical considerations.
2. Provide information to sexually active adolescent and adult males regardless of circumcision status
All sexually active adolescent and adult males should consider using other proven HIV and STI risk-reduction strategies such as reducing the number of partners, correct and consistent use of male latex condoms, and HIV preexposure or postexposure prophylaxis
3. Provide information to uncircumcised sexually active adolescent and adult males
Prior to sharing information about medically performed male circumcision, uncircumcised sexually active adolescent and adult males should be assessed to determine their HIV risk behaviors, HIV infection status, and the gender of their sexual partner(s). These assessments will inform the discussion with men about the risks and benefits of medically performed male circumcision.
3A. Provide information to uncircumcised adolescent and adult males who are heterosexually and bisexually active (i.e., men who have sex with women)
3A-1. Assess the patient's risk of acquiring HIV through heterosexual sex:

• Review the patient's HIV risk behavior
• Assess condom use practices, consistency of use, and barriers to use
• Inform heterosexually and bisexually active adolescent and adult males that males at high risk of HIV exposure during heterosexual sex include HIV uninfected males in sexual relationships with:
   o An HIV-infected woman (i.e., in an HIV discordant couple)
   o One or more females who are at high risk for HIV (this includes commercial sex workers, females who inject drugs, and females in defined geographic locations with a prevalence of HIV >1.0%);
   o Multiple female partners

3A-2. Regardless of assessed risks in 3A-1, all uncircumcised adolescent and adult males who engage in heterosexual sex should be informed about the significant, but partial, efficacy of male circumcision in reducing the risk of acquiring HIV and some STIs through heterosexual sex, as well as the potential harms of male circumcision.
• Male circumcision reduces, but does not eliminate, the risk of acquiring HIV and some STIs during penile-vaginal sex. In clinical trials, medically performed male circumcision reduced the incidence of genital ulcer disease (GUD) by 48% and the prevalence by 47% and reduced the prevalence of HR-HPV by 23%–47% among circumcised men. • Male circumcision has not been shown to reduce the risk of HIV during receptive anal sex. • Male circumcision has not been shown to reduce the risk of STIs during anal sex. • The effect of male circumcision on reducing the risk of HIV and STI transmission during oral sex has not been evaluated • Male circumcision has not been shown to reduce the risk of HIV transmission to female partners. However, in clinical trials, medically performed male circumcision reduced the prevalence of GUD by 22%, HR-HPV by 28%, T. vaginalis by 48%, and bacterial vaginosis by 40% among female partners. • Male circumcision has been shown to reduce the risk of urinary tract infections in males aged 0–1 years by 90%, in males aged 1–16 years by 85%, and in males >16 years by 71%. • During adulthood, uncircumcised males are more likely than circumcised males to experience invasive penile cancer. • After circumcision, men should not have sex until their health care provider has documented wound healing.

Male Circumcision and Infection - Information to Share (continued)
3B. Provide information to men who have sex with men (exclusively)
• Male circumcision reduces the risk of men acquiring HIV and other STIs during penile-vaginal sex, but no definitive statements can be made about whether male circumcision reduces the risk of MSM acquiring HIV and other STIs during penile-anal sex.   • Data pooled across several observational studies indicate that among MSM who practice mainly or exclusively insertive anal sex, circumcision was associated with a decreased risk of acquiring a new HIV infection for the insertive partner; however, numbers of MSM in clinical trials are not enough to make a definitive conclusion.   • It is biologically plausible that MSM who practice mainly insertive anal sex may experience a reduction in the risk for acquiring HIV and STIs like that among heterosexuals in clinical trials during penile-vaginal sex; among men who practice mainly or exclusively receptive-anal sex, male circumcision does not provide a biologically plausible benefit for a similar reduction in risk.
4. Provide information to parents of male newborns, children, or adolescents
Health benefits and risks of elective neonatal, pediatric, or adolescent male circumcision should be considered in consultation with medical providers. Ideally, discussions about neonatal circumcision should occur prior to the birth of the child. Ultimately, whether to circumcise a male neonate or child is a decision made by parents or guardians on behalf of their newborn son or dependent child.
4A. Parents and guardians should be informed about the medical benefits and risks of neonatal, pediatric, or adolescent medically performed male circumcision
• During infancy, circumcised infants are less likely than uncircumcised infants to experience urinary tract infections (UTIs); an estimated 7% of infant males presenting with fever in outpatient clinics and emergency rooms had UTIs, including 20% of uncircumcised febrile infants and 2% of circumcised febrile infants aged younger than 3 months of age   • 32% of uncircumcised males compared with 9% of circumcised males will experience a UTI in their lifetime, suggesting that circumcision is associated with a 23% absolute decreased lifetime risk of UTI   • Although most UTIs are treatable, serious complications may occur when UTIs are not diagnosed, recurrent, difficult to treat, or left untreated. Such complications may include sepsis, pyelonephritis, and renal scarring and have been associated with an increased risk for long-term consequences, including hypertension, build-up of kidney waste products (uremia), and end-stage renal disease   • 8% of annual HIV diagnoses in the United States are among persons with infection attributed to heterosexual contact. STIs are very common, with human papilloma virus (HPV) infection of the anus or genitals occurring in many sexually active persons, although HPV vaccination is highly effective against many serotypes.   • Current risks for either HIV or other non-HIV STIs may not remain constant in the future and the future risk for any individual neonate, child, or adolescent cannot be definitively defined at the time that a circumcision decision is made.

Figure 4.
Male circumcision and infection - information to share adapted from "information for providers to share with male patients and parents regarding male circumcision and the prevention of HIV infection, sexually transmitted infections, and other health outcomes" - division of HIV/AIDS prevention National Center for HIV/AIDS, Viral Hepatitis, STD, and TB Prevention Centers for Disease Control and Prevention.

circumcision is now a recommended strategy for HIV prevention in men in developing nations. By reducing the number of new infections in the population, the resource burden of HIV treatment is lessened, and fewer women and babies are exposed to HIV infection. Nearly 15 million voluntary medical male circumcisions (VMMC) have been performed for HIV prevention in 14 countries of eastern and southern Africa during the decade since WHO and UNAIDS recommended VMMC to be a component of HIV prevention intervention [7, 49]. Swaziland was the first country to introduce national early infant male circumcision (EIMC) into VMMC programming for HIV prevention [86]. It is estimated that these VMMCs will avert over half a million new HIV infections through 2030.

Although MC has not been directly associated with decreases in HIV transmission to female partners, MC has health promotion benefits for women. High-consistency evidence exists that male circumcision protects women against cervical cancer, cervical dysplasia, herpes simplex virus type 2, chlamydia, and syphilis. Even in HIV infected men and women, MC appears to have a role in reducing co-infection with syphilis and STIs such as chlamydia and gonorrhea.

To date, there are no formal programs for MC, whether for VMMC or EIMC in developing countries. However, health care workers in developed and developing countries alike must be prepared to counsel parents that choosing EIMC could have protective benefits ranging from UTIs in infancy to STIs in adulthood. In addition, health care workers must be able to counsel sexually active adolescent and adult males not only on safe sex practices, but that MC may be an option to promote their health or that of their partner [12, 87] (**Figure 4**).

World-wide, male circumcision is an important component in the arsenal of tools to prevent disease. It does not replace but strengthens established approaches to prevent and treat infection e.g. avoidance of risky sexual behaviors, condom use, anti-viral/antibiotic medications, and vaccinations. The role of male circumcision to diminish infections, whether urinary tract or STIs, conserves health resources for those with unpreventable illness and more broadly, can play a role in increasing the health of the population overall.

Author details

Ruth Mielke
California State University Fullerton, Fullerton, California, United States

*Address all correspondence to: ruthmielke@fullerton.edu

IntechOpen

References

[1] Hutchinson J. On the influence of circumcision in preventing syphilis. Boston Medical Surgical Journal. 1856;**55**:77-78

[2] Wolbarst AL. Universal circumcision as a sanitary measure. Journal of the American Medical Association. 1914;**62**(2):92

[3] Auvert B, Taljaard D, Lagarde E, Sobngwi-Tambekou J, Sitta R, Puren A. Randomized, controlled intervention trial of male circumcision for reduction of HIV infection risk: The ANRS 1265 trial. PLoS Medicine. 2005;**2**(11):e298

[4] Bailey R, Moses S, Parker C, Agot K, Maclean I, Krieger J, et al. Male circumcision for HIV prevention in young men in Kisumu, Kenya: A randomised controlled trial. Lancet. 2007;**369**:643-656

[5] Gray R, Kigozi G, Serwadda D, Makumbi F, Watya S, Nalugoda F, et al. Male circumcision for HIV prevention in men in Rakai, Uganda: A randomised trial. Lancet. 2007;**369**:657-666

[6] WHO/UNAIDS. Male Circumcision: Global Trends and Determinants of Prevalence, Safety and Acceptability. Geneva, Switzerland: World Health Organization; 2008

[7] World Health Organization. New Data on Male Circumcision and HIV Prevention: Policy and Programme Implications. Geneva: World Health Organization; 2007

[8] American Urological Association. Circumcision. 2018. Available from: http://www.auanet.org/about/policystatements/circumcision.cfm

[9] Sorokan ST, Finlay JC, Jefferies AL, Canadian Paediatric Society F, Newborn Committee ID, Immunization C. Newborn male circumcision. Paediatrics & Child Health. 2015;**20**(6):311-315

[10] Dave S, Afshar K, Braga LH, Anderson P. Canadian Urological Association guideline on the care of the normal foreskin and neonatal circumcision in Canadian infants (full version). Canadian Urological Association journal (Journal de l'Association des urologues du Canada). 2018;**12**(2):E76

[11] Morris BJ, Wodak AD, Mindel A, Schrieber L, Duggan KA, Dilley A, et al. The 2010 Royal Australasian College of Physicians' policy statement 'circumcision of infant males' is not evidence based. Internal Medicine Journal. 2012;**42**(7):822-828

[12] Centers for Disease Control and Prevention. Information for Providers Counseling Male Patients and Parents Regarding Male Circumcision and the Prevention of HIV Infection, STIs, and Other Health Outcomes. Atlanta, Georgia: Department of Health and Human Services; 2018

[13] American Academy of Pediatrics Task Force on Circumcision. Male Circumcision. Pediatrics. 2012;**130**(3):e756-ee85

[14] Hayashi Y, Kojima Y, Mizuno K, Nakane A, Kamisawa H, Maruyama T, et al. A Japanese view on circumcision: Nonoperative management of normal and abnormal prepuce. Urology. 2010;**76**(1):21-24

[15] Cold CJ, Taylor JR. The prepuce. BJU International. 1999;**83**(S1):34-44

[16] Futaba K, Bowley DM. The foreskin: Problems and pathology. Surgery (Oxford). 2010;**28**(8):387-390

[17] Fleiss PM, Hodges FM, Howe RSV. Immunological functions of the

human prepuce. Sexually Transmitted Infections. 1998;**74**:364-367

[18] Hirbod T, Bailey RC, Agot K, Moses S, Ndinya-Achola J, Murugu R, et al. Abundant expression of HIV target cells and C-type lectin receptors in the foreskin tissue of young Kenyan men. The American Journal of Pathology. 2010;**176**(6):2798-2805

[19] Castellsague X, Bosch F, Munoz N, Meijer C, Shah K, de Sanjose S, et al. Male circumcision, penile human papillomavirus infection, and cervical cancer in female partners. The New England Journal of Medicine. 2002;**346**:1105-1112

[20] Klinglmair G, Pichler R, Zelger B, Dogan H, Becker T, Esterbauer J, et al. Prevalence of the human papillomavirus (HPV) expression of the inner prepuce in asymptomatic boys and men. World Journal of Urology. 2013;**31**(6):1389-1394

[21] Prodger JL, Kaul R. The biology of how circumcision reduces HIV susceptibility: Broader implications for the prevention field. AIDS Research and Therapy. 2017;**14**(1):49

[22] Sheerin NS. Urinary tract infection. Medicine. 2015;**43**(8):435-439

[23] Winberg J, Andersen HJ, Bergström T, Jacobsson B, Larson H, Lincoln K. Epidemiology of symptomatic urinary tract infection in childhood. Acta Paediatrica. 1974;**63**:1-20

[24] Rasouly HM, Lu W. Lower urinary tract development and disease. Wiley Interdisciplinary Reviews. Systems Biology and Medicine. 2013;**5**(3):307-342

[25] Sureshkumar P, Jones M, Cumming RG, Craig JC. Risk factors for urinary tract infection in children: A population-based study of 2856 children. Journal of Paediatrics and Child Health. 2009;**45**(3):87-97

[26] Morris BJ, Wiswell TE. Circumcision and lifetime risk of urinary tract infection: A systematic review and meta-analysis. The Journal of Urology. 2013;**189**(6):2118-2124

[27] To T, Agha M, Dick PT, Feldman W. Cohort study on circumcision of newborn boys and subsequent risk of urinary-tract infection. The Lancet. 1998;**352**(9143):1813-1816

[28] Laway M, Wani M, Patnaik R, Kakru D, Ismail S, Shera A, et al. Does circumcision alter the periurethral uropathogenic bacterial flora. African Journal of Paediatric Surgery. 2012;**9**(2):109-112

[29] Jagannath Vanitha A, Fedorowicz Z, Sud V, Verma Abhishek K, Hajebrahimi S. Routine neonatal circumcision for the prevention of urinary tract infections in infancy. Cochrane Database of Systematic Reviews. 2012;(11). DOI: 10.1002/14651858.CD009129.pub2/abstract

[30] Chesney RW, Carpenter MA, Moxey-Mims M, Nyberg L, Greenfield SP, Hoberman A, et al. Randomized intervention for children with vesicoureteral reflux (RIVUR): Background commentary of RIVUR investigators. Pediatrics. 2008;**122**(Supplement 5):S233-S2S9

[31] Singh-Grewal D, Macdessi J, Craig J. Circumcision for the prevention of urinary tract infection in boys: A systematic review of randomised trials and observational studies. Archives of Disease in Childhood. 2005;**90**(8):853-858

[32] Nguyen HT, Benson CB, Bromley B, Campbell JB, Chow J, Coleman B, et al. Multidisciplinary consensus on the classification of prenatal and postnatal urinary tract dilation (UTD classification system). Journal of Pediatric Urology. 2014;**10**(6):982-998

[33] Braga LH, Farrokhyar F, D'Cruz J, Pemberton J, Lorenzo AJ. Risk factors for febrile urinary tract infection in children with prenatal hydronephrosis: A prospective study. The Journal of Urology. 2015;**193**(5, Supplement):1766-1771

[34] Zaffanello M, Malerba G, Cataldi L, Antoniazzi F, Franchini M, Monti E, et al. Genetic risk for recurrent urinary tract infections in humans: A systematic review. Journal of Biomedicine & Biotechnology. 2010;**2010**:321082

[35] World Health Organization. Report on Global Sexually Transmitted Infection Surveillance. Geneva: WHO; 2018

[36] Rowley J, Vander Hoorn S, Korenromp E, Low N, Unemo M, Abu-Raddad LJ, et al. Global and Regional Estimates of the Prevalence and Incidence of Four Curable Sexually Transmitted Infections in 2016. Geneva, Switzerland: Bulletin of the World Health Organization; 2019. Available from: https://www.who.int/bulletin/online_first/BLT.18.228486.pdf

[37] Kent B. Sexually transmitted bacterial and protozoal infections. Clinical Laboratory Science. 2017;**30**(2):114-119

[38] Katharine JL, Amalia SM, Katherine MET, Peter V, Sami LG, Lori MN. Global estimates of prevalent and incident herpes simplex virus type 2 infections in 2012. PLoS One. 2015;**10**(1):e114989

[39] World Health Organization. HIV/AIDS: Data and Statistics. Geneva, Switzerland: World Health Organization; 2018. Available from: https://www.who.int/hiv/data/en/

[40] Joint United Nations Programme on HIV/AIDS (UNAIDS). UNAIDS Data 2018. Geneva, Switzerland: World Health Organization; 2018. Available from: https://www.unaids.

org/sites/default/files/media_asset/unaids-data-2018_en.pdf

[41] Fink A. A possible explanation for heterosexual male infection with AIDS. The New England Journal of Medicine. 1986;**315**(18):1167

[42] Weiss HA, Quigley MA, Hayes RJ. Male circumcision and risk of HIV infection in sub-Saharan Africa: A systematic review and meta-analysis. AIDS. 2000;**14**(15):2361-2370

[43] Siegfried N, Muller M, Volmink J, Deeks J, Egger M, Low N, et al. Male circumcision for prevention of heterosexual acquisition of HIV in men. Cochrane Database of Systematic Reviews. 2003;**3**:CD003362

[44] Krieger JN. Male circumcision and HIV infection risk. World Journal of Urology. 2012;**30**(1):3-13

[45] Wei Q, Shi B, Lu Y, Lv X, Han P. Circumcision status and risk of HIV acquisition during heterosexual intercourse for both males and females: A meta-analysis. PLoS One. 2015;**10**(5):e0125436

[46] Wawer MJ, Makumbi F, Kigozi G, Serwadda D, Watya S, Nalugoda F, et al. Circumcision in HIV-infected men and its effect on HIV transmission to female partners in Rakai, Uganda: A randomised controlled trial. The Lancet. 2009;**374**(9685):229-237

[47] Grund JM, Bryant TS, Jackson I, Curran K, Bock N, Toledo C, et al. Association between male circumcision and women's biomedical health outcomes: A systematic review. The Lancet Global Health. 2017;**5**(11):e1113-e1e22

[48] Serwadda D, Wawer M, Makumbi F, Kong X, Kigozi G, Gravitt P, et al. Circumcision of HIV-infected men: Effects on high-risk human papillomavirus infections in a

randomized trial in Rakai, Uganda. The Journal of Infectious Diseases. 2010;**201**:1463-1469

[49] World Health Organization. Voluntary Medical Male Circumcision for HIV Prevention in 14 Priority Countries In Eastern and Southern Africa. 2017. Available from: http://www.who.int/hiv/pub/malecircumcision/vmmc-progress-brief-2017

[50] Awad SF, Sgaier SK, Lau FK, Mohamoud YA, Tambatamba BC, Kripke KE, et al. Could circumcision of HIV-positive males benefit voluntary medical male circumcision programs in Africa? Mathematical modeling analysis. PLoS One. 2017;**12**(1):e0170641-e

[51] Nash S DS, Croxford S, Guerra L, Lowndes C, Connor N, Gill ON et al. Progress towards Ending the HIV Epidemic in the United Kingdom: 2018 Report. London: Public Health England; 2018

[52] Centers for Disease Control. HIV/AIDS: Basic Statistics. 2019. Available from: https://www.cdc.gov/hiv/basics/statistics.html

[53] Wiysonge CS, Kongnyuy EJ, Shey M, Muula AS, Navti OB, Akl EA, et al. Male circumcision for prevention of homosexual acquisition of HIV in men. Cochrane Database of Systematic Reviews. 2011;(6):CD007496. DOI: 10.1002/14651858.CD007496.pub2

[54] Sharma SC, Raison N, Khan S, Shabbir M, Dasgupta P, Ahmed K. Male circumcision for the prevention of human immunodeficiency virus (HIV) acquisition: A meta-analysis. BJU International. 2018;**121**(4):515-526

[55] Chelimo C, Wouldes TA, Cameron LD, Elwood JM. Risk factors for and prevention of human papillomaviruses (HPV), genital warts and cervical cancer. The Journal of Infection. 2013;**66**(3):207-217

[56] Hutter JN, Decker CF. Human papillomavirus infection. Disease-a-Month. 2016;**62**(8):294-300

[57] de Sanjosé S, Diaz M, Castellsagué X, Clifford G, Bruni L, Muñoz N, et al. Worldwide prevalence and genotype distribution of cervical human papillomavirus DNA in women with normal cytology: A meta-analysis. The Lancet Infectious Diseases. 2007;**7**(7):453-459

[58] Bray F, Ferlay J, Soerjomataram I, Siegel RL, Torre LA, Jemal A. Global cancer statistics 2018: GLOBOCAN estimates of incidence and mortality worldwide for 36 cancers in 185 countries. CA: A Cancer Journal for Clinicians. 2018;**68**(6):394-424

[59] World Health Organization. Cancer: Cervical cancer. Geneva, Switzerland: World Health Organization; 2018. Available from: https://www.who.int/cancer/prevention/diagnosis-screening/cervical-cancer/en/

[60] Wawer MJ, Tobian AA, Kigozi G, Kong X, Gravitt PE, Serwadda D, et al. Effect of circumcision of HIV-negative men on transmission of human papillomavirus to HIV-negative women: A randomised trial in Rakai, Uganda. The Lancet. 2011;**377**(9761):209-218

[61] Brinton LA, Reeves WC, Brenes MM, Herrero R, Gaitan E, Tenorio F, et al. The male factor in the etiology of cervical cancer among sexually monogamous women. International Journal of Cancer. 1989;**44**(2):199-203

[62] Albero GMPH, Castellsague XP, Giuliano ARP, Bosch FXP. Male circumcision and genital human papillomavirus: A systematic review and meta-analysis. Sexually Transmitted Diseases. 2012;**39**(2):104-113

[63] Larke N, Thomas SL, dos Santos Silva I, Weiss HA. Male circumcision and human papillomavirus infection in men: A systematic review and meta-analysis. The Journal of Infectious Diseases. 2011;**204**(9):1375-1390

[64] Cardona C, Garcia-Perdomo H. Incidence of penile cancer worldwide: Systematic review and meta-analysis. Revista Panamericana de Salud Pública. 2017;**41**:1-10

[65] Minhas S, Manseck A, Watya S, Hegarty PK. Penile cancer—Prevention and premalignant conditions. Urology. 2010;**76**(2 Suppl 1):S24-S35

[66] Freeman EE, Weiss HA, Glynn JR, Cross PL, Whitworth JA, Hayes RJ. Herpes simplex virus 2 infection increases HIV acquisition in men and women: Systematic review and meta-analysis of longitudinal studies. AIDS. 2006;**20**(1):73-83

[67] Tobian A, Charvat B, Ssempijja V, Kigozi G, Serwadda D, Makumbi F, et al. Factors associated with the prevalence and incidence of herpes simplex virus type 2 infection among men in Rakai, Uganda. The Journal of Infectious Diseases. 2009;**199**:945-949

[68] Abu-Raddad LJ, Magaret AS, Celum C, Wald A, Longini IM Jr, Self SG, et al. Genital herpes has played a more important role than any other sexually transmitted infection in driving HIV prevalence in Africa. PLoS One. 2008;**3**(5):e2230-e

[69] Pialoux G, Vimont S, Moulignier A, Buteux M, Abraham B, Bonnard P. Effect of HIV infection on the course of syphilis. AIDS Reviews. 2008;**10**(2):85-92

[70] World Health Organization. Facts Sheets: Herpes Simplex Virus. 2019. Available from: https://www.who.int/news-room/fact-sheets/detail/herpes-simplex-virus

[71] Gantt S, Muller WJ. The immunologic basis for severe neonatal herpes disease and potential strategies for therapeutic intervention. Clinical and Developmental Immunology. 2013;**2013**:16

[72] Looker KJ, Magaret AS, May MT, Turner KME, Vickerman P, Newman LM, et al. First estimates of the global and regional incidence of neonatal herpes infection. The Lancet Global Health. 2017;**5**(3):e300-e3e9

[73] Corey L, Wald A. Maternal and neonatal herpes simplex virus infections. The New England Journal of Medicine. 2009;**361**(14):1376-1385

[74] McQuillan G, Kruszon-Moran D, Flagg EW, Paulose-Ram R. Prevalence of Herpes Simplex Virus Type 1 and Type 2 in Persons Aged 14-49: United States, 2015-2016. Hyattsville, MD: National Center for Health Statistics; 2018

[75] Rajagopal S, Magaret A, Mugo N, Wald A. Incidence of herpes simplex virus type 2 infections in Africa: A systematic review. Open Forum Infectious Diseases. 2014;**1**(2):1-11

[76] Korenromp EL, Rowley J, Alonso M, Mello MB, Wijesooriya NS, Mahiané SG, et al. Global burden of maternal and congenital syphilis and associated adverse birth outcomes-estimates for 2016 and progress since 2012. PLoS One. 2019;**14**(2):e0211720

[77] Taylor M, Newman L, Ishikawa N, Laverty M, Hayashi C, Ghidinelli M, et al. Elimination of mother-to-child transmission of HIV and syphilis (EMTCT): Process, progress, and program integration. PLoS Medicine. 2017;**14**(6):e1002329-e

[78] Centers for Disease Control and Prevention. Sexually Transmitted Disease Surveillance 2017. Atlanta: U.S. Department of Health and Human Services; 2018

[79] Stoltey JE, Cohen SE. Syphilis transmission: A review of the current evidence. Sexual Health. 2015;12(2):103-109

[80] Weiss H, Thomas S, Munabi S, Hayes R. Male circumcision and risk of syphilis, chancroid, and genital herpes: A systematic review and meta-analysis. Sexually Transmitted Infections. 2006;82:101-109

[81] Nayyar C, Chander R, Gupta P, Sherwal BL. Co-infection of human immunodeficiency virus and sexually transmitted infections in circumcised and uncircumcised cases in India. Indian Journal of Sexually Transmitted Diseases and AIDS. 2014;35(2):114-117

[82] Pintye J, Baeten JM, Manhart LE, Celum C, Ronald A, Mugo N, et al. Association between male circumcision and incidence of syphilis in men and women: A prospective study in HIV-1 serodiscordant heterosexual African couples. The Lancet Global Health. 2014;2(11):e664-e671

[83] Yarbrough ML, Burnham C-AD. The ABCs of STIs: An update on sexually transmitted infections. Clinical Chemistry. 2016;62(6):811

[84] Stoner BP, Cohen SE. Lymphogranuloma venereum 2015: Clinical presentation, diagnosis, and treatment: Table 1. Clinical Infectious Diseases. 2015;61(suppl_8):S865-S873

[85] Gray R, Kigozi G, Serwadda D, Makumbi F, Nalugoda F, Watya S, et al. The effects of male circumcision on female partners' genital tract symptoms and vaginal infections in a randomized trial in Rakai, Uganda. American Journal of Obstetrics and Gynecology. 2009;200:e1-e7

[86] Fitzgerald L, Benzerga W, Mirira M, Adamu T, Shissler T, Bitchong R, et al. Scaling up early infant male circumcision: Lessons from the kingdom of Swaziland.

Global Health: Science and Practice. 2016;4(Suppl 1):S76-S86

[87] Mielke RT. Counseling parents who are considering newborn male circumcision. Journal of Midwifery & Women's Health. 2013;58(6):671-682

www.ingramcontent.com/pod-product-compliance
Lightning Source LLC
Chambersburg PA
CBHW081239190326
41458CB00016B/5846